KT-173-729

HIV and Midwifery Practice

Also available in the 'Current Issues in Midwifery' series:

Psychology for Midwives by Ruth Paradice

Health-related Fitness during Pregnancy by Sylvia Baddeley

Obstetric Litigation from A–Z by Andrew Symon

Demystifying Qualitative Research in Pregnancy and Childbirth edited by Tina Lavender, Grace Edwards and Zarko Alfirevic

Perineal Care: An international issue edited by Christine Henderson and Debra Bick

Challenges for Midwives, volume one edited by Yana Richens

Birthing Positions by Regina Coppen

Series editor: Jane Susan Bott

HIV and Midwifery Practice

Jane Susan Bott

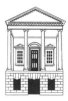

Quay Books
MA Healthcare Limited

Quay Books Division, MA Healthcare Limited, St Jude's Church, Dulwich Road,
London SE24 0PB

British Library Cataloguing-in-Publication Data
A catalogue record is available for this book

© MA Healthcare Limited 2005
ISBN 185642 255 0

Printed in the UK by Cromwell Press, Trowbridge, Wiltshire

Contents

Foreword

Acquired immune deficiency syndrome (AIDS) is a major challenge to healthcare professionals and the wider community. Unless something changes, over 200 million men, women and children will die of AIDS. The epidemic is out of control in the poorest nations, killing four times as many people every week as fifteen years ago. Sadly, a small but significant number of midwives and other healthcare workers are becoming infected in the course of their work. In addition, many babies are needlessly being exposed to risk and are dying later from AIDS as a result of ignorance or lack of access to appropriate treatment including antiviral therapy during pregnancy, avoiding breast-feeding, and so on. And many mothers in different parts of the world are not receiving the right care.

AIDS raises a huge number of complex health and ethical issues which every midwife needs to be aware of. With over eighty-five million already human immunodeficiency virus (HIV)-infected the epidemic is still in the earliest stages. Many parts of Africa are already devastated and history is repeating itself in places like India, China and Russia, on a vast and tragic scale. There is still no vaccine, and no cure, although treatment prolongs life and saves most babies of infected mothers from developing AIDS.

I will never forget the first person I met with AIDS: a young man desperately ill in a hospital side-room. He was anxious, restless, sweaty, fighting for every breath, suffocating in his own secretions and gripped with terrible fear, totally alone and about to die. I was shocked that anyone in a London hospital should be abandoned in such a state. But that's how things were back in 1987, when no hospice in Britain would accept someone with AIDS, when some nurses refused to visit people with AIDS at home and when some of my fellow doctors refused to prescribe appropriate medicines. Fortunately, attitudes and practices have improved enormously, thanks, in no small measure, to huge investment in training and professional education which is what this useful book is all about.

That young man died peacefully, several days later, with the right treatment, and with his loving family by his side, but the whole episode shook me profoundly. I would never be the same again.

Infection rates falling in Uganda

Uganda is a wonderful example of what can happen when governments, companies and non-profit organisations work in partnership, with dramatic falls in infection — from 22% to less than 8% in some groups.

As healthcare professionals we are called to give unconditional compassionate care to all in need, regardless of how they come to be so. Those with AIDS are lepers of today, in many countries facing fear, violence and rejection. It seems incredible today that in the 1980s many UK healthcare workers refused to get involved, and that some people with HIV got beaten up or their homes set on fire because of their diagnosis. Yet the same kind of discrimination and violence still happens in other parts of the world today.

We are in a race against time. We must learn lessons from the past. As we have seen in countries like Uganda, HIV can be beaten, step-by-step, when we all pull together: community organisations, leaders, business, media, schools, churches and government. We must make sure we act fast to save lives — as well as care. Investing in care alone is a disastrous and short-sighted strategy, that will result in deaths of another generation of men, women and children. For the same cost as running a fifty-bed AIDS hospital for a year, we can save up to 10,000 lives, and prevent maybe 50,000 children from bereavement.

After an appallingly slow international response, the wealthiest nations have finally woken up to the nightmare in poorer nations. International agencies, multi-nationals, foundations and governments are now committing far greater resources to fight spread and improve care. But they are severely handicapped by the lack of quality, 'on the ground' community programmes and networks.

It costs almost nothing to save a life or help someone in need. It costs very little to make a huge difference in places like Zimbabwe. Just a couple of pounds a month is enough to help give basic support for a child or adult affected by HIV. And, it costs almost nothing to save a life: to talk about the illness and keep it on the agenda in a way that encourages people to change the way they live.

As a UK midwife it costs nothing to take a little extra time with a mother who has HIV who is worried about her future and that of her child. It costs nothing to talk about HIV in antenatal clinics and ask the difficult but important questions.

Dr Patrick Dixon
March 2005

Dr Patrick Dixon is author of *The Truth about AIDS* and Founder of Aids Care Education and Training (ACET) International Alliance, a community of independent agencies providing AIDS care and prevention programmes in many countries, in partnership with local churches of different denominations.

Dixon P (1994) *The Truth about Aids*. Kingsway, Eastbourne. Available online:
   http://www.acet-international.org

Introduction

My interest in human immunodeficiency virus (HIV) began when I heard Dr Patrick Dixon speak at a conference. He had been working as a medical doctor caring for people with HIV/acquired immune deficiency syndrome (AIDS). Having encountered first hand the problems facing people affected by HIV/AIDS, he went on to set up a voluntary organisation in 1988, known as ACET (Aids Care Education and Training). This has expanded over the years into a global network (ACET International Alliance), providing sexual health and drugs education, home-based and in-patient AIDS care, housing support, income generation projects, orphan support, bereavement support, professional training and technical advice in communities across many nations on issues relating to HIV/AIDS.

This interest began to influence my professional development, and I undertook the post-registration module 'caring for people with HIV/AIDS'. At that time, HIV screening was being offered to selected pregnant women, mainly in London. I subsequently undertook a Master of Science degree in Midwifery Studies, which enabled me to focus in more depth. This included being able to discuss critically gender issues, particularly related to HIV screening in practice, and to explore interprofessional collaboration, including voluntary sector services, to meet the needs of HIV-infected women and their families.

I also undertook qualitative research on the adoption of universal precautions in midwifery practice, which was completed in 1997. I then agreed to write a series of six articles for the *British Journal of Midwifery*. While I was working on these articles, the Department of Health (DoH) issued a press release publicising new guidelines requiring midwives to offer and recommend HIV screening to all women during pregnancy. I introduced the series with an 'editorial' in November 1999, highlighting some of the issues for midwives related to implementing a universal screening policy. These articles were used as a basis for the chapters in this book.

I have worked in midwifery education over the past fourteen years, and my role as senior lecturer at Kingston University and St George's Hospital Medical School has given me the impetus to write this book, as a midwife, for midwives. The contents are relevant to all those involved in maternity care provision, including midwives, student midwives, midwifery managers and midwifery educationalists. The book provides the reader with a current perspective on HIV, including recent statistics, research evidence for clinical excellence and DoH guidelines of relevance to midwifery practice.

Midwives are required to practice in a constantly changing society. Increasing HIV prevalence rates are being reported each year, both globally and nationally. Heterosexual transmission is the primary mode of HIV infection worldwide, and the majority of HIV-infected pregnant women in the United Kingdom were born in sub-Saharan Africa. The devastating impact of HIV/ AIDS, in addition to reducing life expectancy, is associated with deepening poverty, most notably in sub-Saharan Africa. An understanding of the HIV epidemic and its impact, both nationally and globally, will enable midwives to provide effective pre-conception care, and care during pregnancy, labour and the postnatal period. Some of the challenges facing midwives are:

⌘ HIV screening during pregnancy — reducing the risk of mother to child transmission to below 2% with targeted interventions.
⌘ Professional issues, eg. maintaining confidentiality.
⌘ Meeting the needs of vulnerable groups, eg. asylum seekers.
⌘ Understanding cultural issues when providing care in partnership with HIV-infected women.
⌘ Understanding the psychological and social impact of HIV, eg. fear, rejection, isolation, loss of income, stigma and discrimination, and minimising harm where possible.
⌘ Public health issues — health promotion.
⌘ Infection control — reducing the risk of occupational infection.

This book enables readers to develop their understanding and practice when providing effective care to HIV-infected women and their families, and to function effectively within an interprofessional team. Effective interprofessional collaboration is associated with the provision of a seamless service, which ultimately benefits patients. Ideally, midwives should be able to provide continuity of midwifery care (named midwife) throughout the pregnancy, labour and postnatal period, working collaboratively with paediatricians, HIV physicians and obstetricians. The book helps readers to recognise the special needs of HIV-infected women and their families, and to provide care that is sensitive to those needs. For example, the need to protect confidentiality, and to make referrals to other sources of support, such as counsellors, social workers and voluntary organisations/support groups. It is hoped that this book will develop readers' understanding of health promotion and disease prevention in relation to HIV infection. Such knowledge will assist midwives in facilitating informed decision making by women to reduce the risk of HIV transmission and minimise the potentially harmful effects of HIV.

The book is divided into six chapters. *Chapter 1* provides the reader with an understanding of the structure of the virus, the routes of transmission, disease progression and an overview of the global and national spread of HIV. *Chapter 2* will enable readers to appreciate the effect of HIV on women's health, and the management and care of women who are infected. *Chapter 3* offers an understanding of ethical principles and their application to midwifery practice.

Beneficence, non-maleficence, autonomy, informed consent and confidentiality are discussed in relation to offering and recommending HIV screening during pregnancy. *Chapter 4* includes further discussion of HIV screening, focusing in particular on gender issues related to sexual health promotion and reduction of mother to child transmission. *Chapter 5* provides readers with an understanding of the need to prevent occupationally-acquired HIV infection, the problems and barriers to adopting universal precautions in midwifery practice and factors that motivate and support midwives to adopt universal precautions. I have included my research, which assesses and develops the practice of midwives in relation to the adoption of universal precautions. This chapter is relatively detailed and includes a literature review, research methodology, discussion of my research findings and recommendations. Finally, *Chapter 6* provides further discussion of health and safety issues for midwives, including protection of clients from HIV-infected healthcare workers.

Jane Susan Bott
January, 2005

Acknowledgements

This book is the culmination of much work over the past ten years, reflecting my interest in HIV and, in particular, its relevance for midwifery practice. I would like to thank Jill Stewart-Moore, Teaching Fellow (Midwifery), School of Nursing and Midwifery, Queen's University Belfast, who was instrumental in helping me to gain a good knowledge base in the care of people with HIV and AIDS. I would also like to thank Carolyn Roth, Lecturer in Midwifery at City University, for her help and support while I was undertaking my research into the adoption of universal precautions in midwifery practice. In addition, I would like to thank Val Collington, Deputy Dean, Kingston University and St George's, University of London, for supporting my professional development.

I would also like to thank the midwives who participated in the focus group discussions, and Valerie Sheridan, Acting Head of the School of Midwifery, Kingston University and St George's, University of London, who acted as assistant moderator for my research. My gratitude goes also to the midwifery managers who agreed to be interviewed, the head of midwifery who gave me permission to take photographs for the purpose of my research, and the people who were photographed.

I would like to thank Binkie (former publisher of Quay Books) who has been very encouraging and supportive, and has worked hard to ensure the book goes to press.

This is a book about challenges. I faced my own challenge three years ago when I was diagnosed with breast cancer. I would like to thank Dr Maryse Desor (my GP), and Mr Graham Layer, Dr Anthony Neal and the breast cancer care team at The Royal Surrey County Hospital for all their support and care. In addition, I would like to thank all my Bosom Buddies who have made life such fun. Without these people I may never have written this book.

Finally, I would like to thank my family for all their love and support. In particular, I would like to thank my parents who have been a constant source of support and encouragement to me throughout my career, and for my wonderful husband, Alan, who has proof read my work and supported me in achieving my dreams.

Chapter 1

HIV modes of spread: a global and national perspective

Human immunodeficiency virus (HIV) poses many challenges, including some that are relevant to midwifery. This chapter will enable midwives to understand the structure of the virus, how infection is transmitted, and the nature of the disease. The emerging pattern of the HIV/acquired immune deficiency syndrome (AIDS) epidemic will be examined from global and national perspectives. The impact of the epidemic will also be considered, highlighting potential areas of concern, global challenges, and some of the immediate challenges across the UK, with reference to the midwife's role where appropriate.

HIV is a fairly complex virus (Heaphy, 1999) which belongs to a group of viruses known as retroviruses (Pratt, 1995). Retroviruses differ from most organisms in that their genetic building blocks consist of ribonucleic acid (RNA) as opposed to deoxyribonucleic acid (DNA) (Toebe, 1999). A retrovirus is able to make a DNA copy of its RNA genetic material. This is made possible by the existence of a special enzyme called reverse transcriptase (Toebe, 1999). HIV is therefore able to make copies of its own genome, as DNA, in host cells such as the human CD4 'helper' lymphocytes (Adler, 1997).

HIV infection results in progressive depletion of the immune system as the virus infects mainly CD4 cells and macrophages. The virus destroys or impairs the function of the infected cells, causing 'immune deficiency'. A deficient immune system is unable to fight off infection and cancers, and so sufferers are more prone to infections such as *pneumocystis carinii* pneumonia, toxoplasmosis, systemic and oesophageal candidiasis, generalised herpes zoster, cryptococcal meningitis, and to cancers such as Kaposi's sarcoma (UNAIDS, 2004a). These diseases are known as 'opportunistic infections' because they take advantage of a weakened immune system.

AIDS was initially defined in 1982, following the first citing of unusual immune system failure among homosexual men in the United States in 1981. HIV was isolated and identified in 1983/84 (UNAIDS, 2004a). Two types of HIV have been identified, namely HIV-1 and HIV-2. Both are transmitted by sexual contact, through blood transfusion, and from mother to child, and both cause AIDS, although HIV-2 seems to be less transmissible and less pathogenic as the period between initial infection and illness is longer (UNAIDS, 2004a).

Structure of HIV

HIV has an outer layer, called the envelope, which it picks up from the host cell membrane as it buds out from the host cell (Toebe, 1999). Numerous spikes with knobs project from the envelope, consisting of protein molecules called gp41 and gp120 respectively (*Figure 1.1*). These glycoproteins are able to bind to receptors on the cells of the immune system which carry a marker, known as the CD4 molecule (Toebe, 1999). The genetic material of HIV is enclosed in a protein coat, known as a capsid, or p24 (Toebe, 1999). The capsid environment contains viral proteins, including reverse transcriptase (Heaphy, 1999). The capsid is surrounded by a layer of matrix protein (MA), or p17 (Heaphy, 1999).

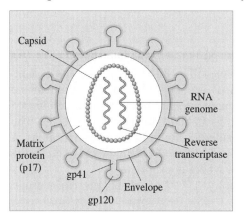

Figure 1.1: Schematic representation of HIV

The gp41 protein enables HIV to fuse with the cell membrane of the host cell. The viral enzymes and RNA are then able to enter the host cell. Reverse transcriptase copies the RNA into DNA, which then integrates into the host cell (School of Medical Sciences, Otago University, 1998). Because the virus copies the CD4 cell's DNA, it cannot be identified and destroyed by the body's defence mechanisms. Virus particles remain in the CD4 cells until their replication is triggered. Then new virus particles emerge from the surface of the CD4 cells in large numbers, destroying the cell in the process. The viruses are then able to infect other cells (UNAIDS, 2004a).

When a person initially becomes infected, there is a burst of activity as many cells are infected and the immune system produces large numbers of antibodies. Although the viral load is high, the person's HIV status cannot be determined using standard blood tests because sufficient numbers of antibodies have not yet been formed. Known as 'the window period', this period lasts from several weeks to months. A person is highly infectious during this time, and will commonly experience a 'flu-like' illness at the end of the window period (UNAIDS, 2004a).

Disease progression

Most people who become infected with HIV will develop signs of AIDS within eight to ten years if they do not receive treatment. However, the course of HIV infection and the development of AIDS does vary. For example, about 5%–10% of HIV-positive individuals develop AIDS symptoms very rapidly during the first years of infection, and about the same proportion remain infected with HIV for fifteen years or more without progressing to AIDS. Symptoms of AIDS generally appear when the CD4 white blood cells fall to 200 per mm^3 of blood (UNAIDS, 2004a).

Prior to the development of HIV viral load testing, CD4 counts and clinical disease parameters were used to assess disease progression. These parameters remain useful clinically, but plasma viral load is now seen as being the single strongest predictor of subsequent CD4 decline and progression to AIDS or death. Different phases of the disease have been identified as follows (Pratt, 1995).

Acute primary infection

Two to four weeks after the initial infection, 40%–60% of people develop acute 'glandular fever-like symptoms'. Symptoms include lethargy and malaise, headache, fever, painful joints, muscular pain, diarrhoea and faintly erythematous skin rashes. Some people may develop aseptic meningitis, encephalitis, and swollen lymph glands (lymphadenopathy). Other people, however, may have unrecognisable symptoms. Towards the end of this phase, HIV antibodies are produced and this is referred to as 'seroconversion'.

Phase B: Antibody positive phase

Following seroconversion, infected people are found to be antibody positive when their blood is tested. During this phase, many people remain clinically asymptomatic.

Phase C: Early symptomatic disease

During this phase, people usually become chronically ill, and may be affected by a variety of minor opportunistic infections such as oral candidiasis.

Phase D: Late symptomatic disease (AIDS)

Patients with AIDS commonly present with a host of opportunistic infections, as various pathogens are able to take the 'opportunity' of a depressed immune system to establish clinical illness.

Phase E: Periods of remission

Treatment of opportunistic infections results in periods of remission and relatively good health.

Phase F: Terminal phase

Pneumocystis carinii pneumonia is a common cause of death. Patients are frequently blind, (because of cytomegalovirus retinitis), incontinent, grossly malnourished and may suffer from dementia.

HIV transmission

Although HIV has been isolated in various body fluids including saliva, tears, urine and cerebrospinal fluid, not all body fluids transmit the virus because of the varying amounts of virus present. Blood, semen and possibly cervical secretions are particularly infectious (Adler, 1997). HIV cannot be transmitted by air, water or casual contact (UNAIDS, 2004a).

Categories of transmission have been identified as follows (Pratt, 1995):

⌘ Drug use.
⌘ Sexual transmission.
⌘ Vertical transmission, ie. during pregnancy, delivery, or breast-feeding. The risk of transmission is 15%–30% in non-breastfed babies. Breast-feeding increases the risk by 10%–15% (UNAIDS, 2004a).
⌘ Iatrogenic transmission, ie. transfusion of blood or blood products, organ or tissue transplant, HIV-contaminated equipment during invasive procedures, occupational infection, or artificial insemination.

Contamination with infected blood through blood transfusion or injecting drugs is the most efficient way of transmitting HIV, although sexual transmission is the predominant mode of transmission (UNAIDS, 2004a). There is a slight risk of HIV transmission when people engage in oral sex, especially when they have abrasions in the mouth or gum disease (UNAIDS, 2004a).

Several factors have been associated with an increased or decreased risk of sexual transmission (*Table 1.1*). For example, anal intercourse carries a greater risk than vaginal intercourse for the receptive partner, and lesions caused by rough sex and rape increase the probability of HIV transmission. In addition, people with untreated sexually transmitted infections (STIs), particularly involving ulcers or discharge, are six to ten times more likely to pass on or acquire HIV during sex. The reason for this is that STIs increase the likelihood of broken skin or membranes allowing the virus to enter or leave the body. Furthermore, the cells that the virus is seeking to infect will be concentrated at the site of the STI because these cells are fighting the STI (UNAIDS, 2004a).

Table 1.1: Factors associated with an increased/decreased risk of sexual transmission (UNAIDS, 2004a)	
Increased risk of HIV transmission	**Decreased risk of HIV transmission**
❖ Anal intercourse compared with vaginal intercourse for the receptive partner	❖ Vaginal intercourse compared with anal intercourse for the receptive partner
❖ If the man is uncircumcised	❖ Male circumcision — very strong — though not conclusive evidence
❖ Lesions caused by rough sex and rape	❖ Gentle sex
❖ Untreated sexually transmitted infections (STIs)	❖ No STIs
❖ If the vagina is immature, eg. in teenage girls	❖ If the vagina is mature, eg. in fully grown women
❖ If the woman is menstruating	❖ If the woman is not menstruating
❖ During acute primary infection phase and during the later phase of HIV disease when the infected person has a very high viral load	❖ During antibody positive phase, when the infected person is clinically asymptomatic

Diagnosing and monitoring HIV infection

Diagnostic tests are becoming cheaper and easier to use in practice. Decision-making diagnosis guidelines have been developed, combining screening tests with high sensitivity, followed by confirmatory tests with high specificity. More information on HIV diagnostics is available online: http://www.who.int/bct/.

Standard techniques for diagnosing HIV infection rely on the detection of antibody responses rather than detection of the virus itself. The two most widely used tests are the enzyme-linked immunosorbent assay (ELISA) and the Western blot, which, combined, have a high sensitivity and specificity (>99%) (Perez *et al*, 2001).

However, the positive predictive value of the two tests, even when used in combination, depends on the characteristics of the population being tested.

For example, if the prevalence of HIV infection is high, as it would be if intravenous drug users from inner cities were tested, the probability that an individual with a positive test is truly infected remains at 100% even when the joint false-positive rate is 0.5%. Conversely, if the prevalence of HIV infection is very low (0.01%), even a joint false-positive rate of 0.02% will mean that at least half of the people who test positive will have a false-positive result.

The most commonly used methods for quantifying viral infection by detecting viral RNA are the polymerase chain reaction (PCR)-based assays and the bDNA assay. Viral load as measured by these techniques is a marker of ongoing HIV viral replication and is a strong predictor of disease progression to AIDS or death (Ho, 1996). Current treatments, referred to as Highly Active Antiretroviral Therapy (HAART) because a combination of different antiretroviral drugs are administered, are effective in controlling virus replication in most patients, reducing the HIV viral load in their blood (UNAIDS, 2004a). Consequently, many more people are able to survive longer, providing they have access to such treatment.

Global perspective

Information on the global AIDS epidemic is published annually and is available online from the UNAIDS website. The *2004 Report on the Global AIDS Epidemic* states that by the end of December 2003, approximately 37.8 million people were living with HIV. It is estimated that 4.8 million of these were newly infected in 2003 (*Figure 1.2*). The number of new infections in 2003 is the greatest number recorded in any one year since the epidemic began. Since 1981, when the first AIDS cases were reported, 20 million people have died, including 2.9 million who died in 2003. *Figures 1.3–1.6* show that some countries are more affected than others. There are also wide regional variations in infection rates (UNAIDS, 2004b).

An estimated 25 million people are reported to be living with HIV in sub-Saharan Africa. The HIV prevalence rates appear to be stabilising, mainly because there has been a rise in AIDS deaths accompanying a continued increase in new infections. However, the prevalence is still rising in some countries, for example in Swaziland, and is declining in others, for example in Uganda. Over 10% of the world's population live in sub-Saharan Africa, and almost two-thirds of all people living with HIV live in sub-Saharan Africa, reflecting the scale of the epidemic in this part of the world. An estimated three million people in sub-Saharan Africa became newly infected in 2003. In addition, 2.2 million died, which represents 75% of the three million AIDS deaths globally that year (UNAIDS, 2004b).

Number of people living with HIV in 2003	Total	37.8 million (34.6–42.3 million)
	Adults	35.7 million (32.7–39.8 million)
	Children under 15 years	2.1 million (1.9 –2.5 million)
People newly infected with HIV in 2003	Total	4.8 million (4.2–6.3 million)
	Adults	4.1 million (3.6–5.6 million)
	Children under 15 years	630,000 (570,000–740,000)
AIDS deaths in 2003	Total	2.9 million (2.6–3.3 million)
	Adults	2.4 million (2.2–2.7 million)
	Children under 15 years	490,000 (440,000–580,000)

Figure 1.2: Global summary of the HIV and AIDS epidemic, December 2003

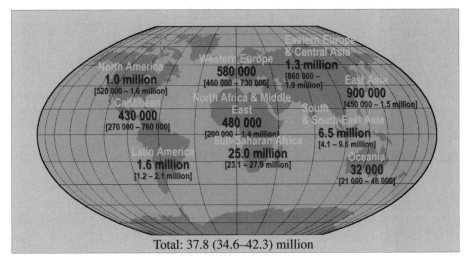

Figure 1.3: Adults and children estimated to be living with HIV, from the end of 2003

There are wide variations in HIV prevalence across Africa. For example, in southern Africa, all seven countries have prevalence rates above 17%. Indeed, Botswana and Swaziland have prevalence rates of over 35%. West Africa has the lowest prevalence, with all countries having a prevalence of below 10%, and most having a prevalence of between 1%–5%. The prevalence in central and east Africa falls somewhere between these two groups, ranging from 4%–13%. An estimated 480,000 people are living with HIV in North Africa and the Middle East, although systematic surveillance of the epidemic is not well developed here, particularly among injecting drug users. In addition, the detection of HIV infection among men who have homosexual sex is problematic, as this practice is widely condemned and illegal in many places (UNAIDS, 2004b).

	Adults and children living with HIV	Adults and children newly-infected with HIV	Adult prevalence rate (%)	Adult and child deaths due to AIDS
Sub-Saharan Africa	25.0 million (23.1–27.9 million)	3.0 million (2.6–3.7 million)	7.5 (6.9–8.3)	2.2 million (2.0–2.5 million)
North Africa and Middle East	480,000 (200,000–1.4 million)	75,000 (21,000–310,000)	0.2 (0.1–0.6)	24,000 (9,900–62,000)
South and South-East Asia	6.5 million (4.1–9.6 million)	850,000 (430,000–2.0 million)	0.6 (0.4–0.9)	460,000 (290,000–700,000)
East Asia	900 000 450,000–1.5 million)	200,000 (62,000–590,000)	0.1 (0.1–0.2)	44,000 (22,000–75,000)
Latin America	1.6 million (1.2–2.1 million)	200,000 (140,000–340,000)	0.6 (0.5–0.8)	84,000 (65,000–110,000)
Caribbean	430,000 (270,000–760,000)	52,000 (26,000–140,000)	2.3 (1.4–4.1)	35,000 (23,000–59,000)
Eastern Europe and Central Asia	1.3 million (860,000–1.9 million)	360 000 (160,000–900,000)	0.6 (0.4–0.9)	49,000 (32,000–71,000)
Western Europe	580 000 (460,000–730,000)	20,000 (13,000–37,000)	0.3 (0.2–0.4)	6,000 (<8 000)
North America	1.0 million (520 000–1.6 million)	44,000 (16,000–120,000)	0.6 (0.3–1.0)	16,000 (8,300–25,000)
Oceania	32,000 (21,000–46,000)	5,000 (2,100–13,000)	0.2 (0.1–0.3)	700 (<1 300)
Total	**37.8 million (34.6–42.3 million)**	**4.8 million (4.2–6.3 million)**	**1.1% (1.0–1.2%)**	**2.9 million (2.6–3.3 million)**

Figure 1.4: Regional HIV and AIDS statistics and features, end of 2003

Because African women become infected at an earlier age than men, they are potentially more at risk. This is borne out in the UNAIDS Report on the global AIDS epidemic (2004b). For example, on average, there are thirteen infected women for every ten infected men. The difference is even more pronounced among fifteen to twenty-four-year-olds, ranging from twenty women for every ten men in South Africa, to forty-five women for every ten men in Kenya and Mali (UNAIDS, 2004b).

The rapid expansion of the epidemic in Asia is mainly attributable to sharp increases in HIV infections in China, Indonesia and Vietnam. It is estimated that 7.4 million people are living with HIV in the region and 1.1 million people became newly infected in 2003, more than in previous years. As 60% of the world's population live in Asia, the global implications of this fast-growing Asian epidemic are immense. The Asian epidemic is largely concentrated among injecting drug users, men who have homosexual sex, sex workers, clients of sex workers and their immediate sexual partners. Stigma and discrimination hamper effective prevention efforts. However, countries such as Thailand and Cambodia, which have chosen to tackle openly high-risk behaviour, such as sex work, have been more successful in fighting HIV, as reflected in the reduced infection rates among sex workers (UNAIDS, 2004b).

Injecting drug use fuels the expanding epidemic in Eastern Europe and Central Asia. Estonia, Latvia, the Russian Federation and Ukraine are the worst affected countries. About 1.3 million people are living with HIV, compared with about 160,000 in 1995. More than 80% of those infected are under the age of thirty (UNAIDS, 2004b).

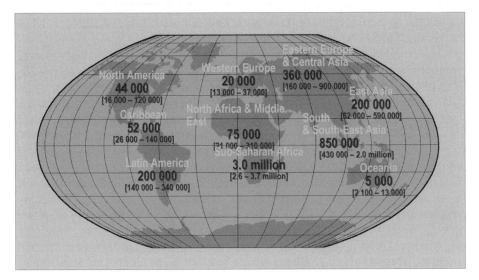

Figure 1.5: Estimated number of adults and children newly-infected with HIV and AIDS during 2003

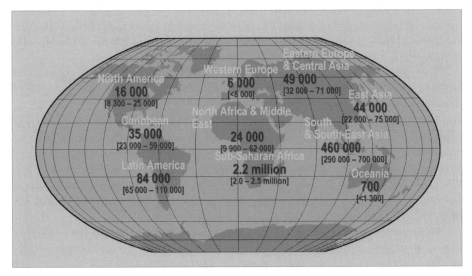

Figure 1.6: Estimated adult and child deaths from AIDS during 2003

In Latin America it is estimated that about 1.6 million people are living with HIV. The groups mostly affected are injecting drug users and men who have homosexual sex. Despite the national prevalence being low in some countries, local epidemics may be problematic. For example, in Brazil, the national prevalence is below 1%, but in certain cities 60% of injecting drug users are infected with HIV (UNAIDS, 2004b).

Around 430,000 people living in the Caribbean are infected with HIV. The main mode of spread is heterosexual, and in many places it is concentrated among sex workers. Haiti has the highest national prevalence of 5.6%, which is the highest outside Africa (UNAIDS, 2004b).

An estimated 1.6 million people are living with HIV in high-income countries, where antiretroviral therapy is available to most people who need it. With treatment, HIV-infected people are able to stay healthy and survive longer than infected people elsewhere in the world. The number of people who are infected with HIV is therefore rising in the USA and in Western Europe. In the USA, an estimated 950,000 people are living with HIV, compared with 900,000 in 2001, and in Western Europe, 580,000 people are living with HIV compared with 540,000 in 2001 (UNAIDS, 2004b).

The devastating impact of AIDS is most apparent in sub-Saharan Africa. In addition to reducing life expectancy, AIDS is associated with deepening poverty, and has contributed to and exacerbated food shortages. As there are no large-scale treatment programmes, and if current infection rates continue, it is predicted that up to 60% of fifteen-year-olds living in the worst affected countries of eastern and southern Africa will not reach their sixtieth birthday. Indeed, the average life expectancy is predicted to fall to below thirty-five years in Swaziland, Zambia and Zimbabwe, without antiretroviral programmes.

However, the availability of antiretroviral treatment would change the future for many people. Statistics show that for people living in low- and middle-income countries, mortality rates among fifteen to forty-nine-year-olds are up to twenty times greater than mortality rates for people living with HIV in industrialised countries (UNAIDS, 2004b).

The impact of HIV on women is particularly evident as they bear the brunt of the burden of caring for sick family members. Young girls are often prevented from attending school because they are required to care for sick parents or younger siblings. Older women often take on the burden of caring for their adult children when they become sick, and when eventually the person dies, the older parents will take on the parenting of the orphaned children. Often they are also responsible for working to provide the family income or the food crops. Because of AIDS-related stigma and discrimination, HIV-infected women are frequently rejected, or they may have their property seized following the death of their husband (UNAIDS, 2004b).

Families affected by AIDS are more likely to suffer severe poverty compared with non-affected households, as sick members of the family are no longer able to work and the family income is reduced. Medical expenses and funeral costs further deplete the family budget. It has been estimated that such expenses use up approximately one-third of the family's income (UNAIDS, 2004b).

In many countries, the AIDS epidemic is intensifying chronic food shortages among large numbers of people who are already undernourished. As a result of AIDS deaths, there is often a reduced agricultural workforce, as well as a reduced family income for buying food. This is a particular problem for people living with AIDS, as they need more calories than uninfected people do. It is believed that AIDS will have claimed the lives of 20% or more of agricultural workers in southern Africa by 2020 (UNAIDS, 2004b).

Globally, AIDS is reducing the prospect of children achieving universal access to primary education by 2015. For example, in countries such as Kenya, Uganda, Swaziland, Zambia and Zimbabwe, the quality of education is suffering as skilled teachers fall sick and die. Many of these countries cannot afford to train more teachers. In addition, children from AIDS-affected families are frequently prevented from attending school as a result of being unable to afford school fees because of a parent's sickness and related expenses, or because they are required to care for sick relatives (UNAIDS, 2004b).

Finally, AIDS is placing an increasing burden on weakened health services. In African countries, for example, it is estimated that AIDS causes 19%–53% of all government health employee deaths. The epidemic is outstripping growth in the supply of healthcare workers (UNAIDS, 2004b).

Global HIV prevention efforts

Fewer than one in five of the world's population have access to HIV prevention services. It has been estimated that if such services were made universally available, 29 million of the 45 million new infections projected to occur this decade could be averted. Key aspects of the UNAIDS (2004b) comprehensive HIV prevention strategy are identified in *Table 1.2*.

In particular, prevention programmes are not reaching the people who need them most. Vulnerable groups include women and young people. To prevent high infection rates among women, the root causes of their vulnerability, including legal, social and economic disadvantages, must be addressed. Young people must have access to knowledge and confidential health information, preventative education and condoms. In countries where preventative programmes have been successful, notably Brazil, the Dominican Republic, Uganda and Thailand, HIV infection rates have fallen (UNAIDS, 2004b).

HIV prevention should be responsive to changing needs. For example, in high-income countries new infections are rising again, particularly among young men who have homosexual sex. This has been attributed to what has been termed 'prevention fatigue' and complacency associated with the availability of antiretroviral treatment (UNAIDS, 2004b).

Expanding the availability of antiretroviral therapies and other treatments should strengthen prevention efforts by encouraging many more people to undergo HIV testing. At present, the proportion of people who would benefit from testing and who are able to have the test ranges from almost none in south-east Asia to 7% in sub-Saharan Africa, and 1.5% in eastern Europe. Where services do exist, fear of stigma and discrimination discourages people from having the test (UNAIDS, 2004b).

Table 1.2: UNAIDS global and HIV prevention strategy

❖   AIDS education and awareness

❖   Behaviour change programmes especially for young people and populations at higher risk of HIV exposure, as well as for people living with HIV

❖   Promoting male and female condoms as a protective option along with abstinence, fidelity and reducing the number of sexual partners

❖   Voluntary counselling and testing

❖   Preventing and treating STIs

❖   Primary prevention among pregnant women and prevention of mother-to-child transmission

❖   Harm reduction programmes for injecting drug users

❖   Measures to protect blood supply safety

❖   Infection control in healthcare settings

❖   Community education and changes in laws and policies to counter stigma and discrimination

❖   Vulnerability reduction through social, legal and economic change

---

Clearly, there is tremendous scope for improvement. New policies need to be implemented that will effectively reduce the vulnerability of large numbers of people. Improvements include access to education, empowerment of women and international cooperation to prevent human trafficking for sexual exploitation. In addition, the 'prevention gap', in which less than one in five people had access to HIV prevention services in 2004, needs closing. HIV prevention should be comprehensive and include a variety of interventions (*Table 1.2*). Individual rights should be protected and AIDS-related stigma and discrimination should be eliminated through effective legal frameworks. In particular, men who have homosexual sex account for 5%–10% of all HIV cases worldwide, and this group is highly stigmatised throughout much of the world. Indeed, eighty-four countries in 2002 had legal prohibitions against sex between men, and this hampers prevention efforts (UNAIDS, 2004b).

Globally, some improvements are being made in providing treatment, care and support for people living with HIV. However, much still needs to be achieved. The World Health Organization (WHO) estimates that nine out of ten people who urgently need HIV treatment are not getting it. Over the next two years, an estimated five to six million people will die if they do not receive antiretroviral treatment. Most countries with national AIDS plans have now set antiretroviral treatment coverage targets. At the same time, the price of antiretroviral medicine has fallen dramatically in many countries (UNAIDS, 2004b).

Countries with antiretroviral medicine manufacturing capacity, for example, Brazil, India and Thailand, are increasingly cooperating with those African countries that wish to set up local production facilities. In addition, some developing countries are working with industrialised countries in Europe and North America, to jointly undertake antiretroviral production technology transfer to developing countries that are interested and able to produce the medicines locally (UNAIDS, 2004b).

Further initiatives are required to provide greater support for technology transfer and exports from countries with antiretroviral manufacturing capacity to countries that lack this provision. Furthermore, national policies and programmes should be agreed and implemented to ensure fair access to treatment. Global funding is also required to meet the needs of all of the world's population. Two-thirds of this funding is expected to come from the international community. Most of the money will be used to meet the needs of the poorest and worst affected countries of Asia and sub-Saharan Africa. These countries will rely on external donors to meet up to 80% of their needs (UNAIDS, 2004b).

UK perspective

The Health Protection Agency publishes annual reports, which provide readers with information on HIV in the UK. These reports are also available online. The report, *Renewing the Focus,* includes national surveillance data for HIV/AIDS and other STIs. It gives an overview of recent trends and highlights potential areas of concern. An increasing incidence and prevalence of HIV and other STIs has been reported, highlighting the immediate public health challenges across the UK (Health Protection Agency, 2003a).

By the end of 2002, an estimated 49,500 adults aged over fifteen were living with HIV in the UK. Of these, 34,300 were diagnosed, and 15,200 were undiagnosed. During 2002, the overall prevalence of HIV infection in adults increased by 20% among those who were diagnosed and by 17% among those who remained undiagnosed. This rise in the overall prevalence has been reported to be mainly due to the possible expansion of HIV transmission in homo/bisexual men and continued migration of HIV-infected heterosexual men and women from sub-Saharan Africa. However, the vast majority of heterosexuals born in sub-Saharan Africa are uninfected. For example, 90% of GUM clinic attendees and 98% of pregnant women surveyed in 2002 were uninfected (Health Protection Agency, 2003a).

The total of 5542 diagnoses in 2002 was almost double the 2814 diagnoses in 1998. Heterosexually-acquired infections are a major component of this recent increase in new HIV diagnoses. This is reflected in the three-fold increase in the number of new heterosexually-acquired infections diagnosed, from less than 900 in 1996 to over 3152 in 2002 (*Figure 1.7*). In 2002, two-thirds of the heterosexually acquired infections newly diagnosed were in women, and over 2300 were in heterosexual men and women born in sub-Saharan Africa. During 1993–1999, HIV infections from east Africa predominated. However, since 1999, infections acquired in south-eastern Africa, particularly Zimbabwe, have dominated (*Figure 1.8*). There has also been a steady increase, over the past five years, in the number of HIV diagnoses in people who are thought to have acquired their infection heterosexually while living in the UK, from 147 in 1998 to 275 reported so far for 2002. The majority of these people were probably infected by partners who acquired their infections outside Europe. Since 1999, the number of newly diagnosed heterosexuals has exceeded the number of newly diagnosed homo/bisexual men (*Figure 1.7*) (Health Protection Agency, 2003a).

The number of new diagnoses of HIV infection acquired through sex between men has been increasing since 1999. In 2001, 1714 diagnoses were reported, which was the largest annual total for ten years. In 2002, 1617 new HIV diagnoses were reported, and this figure will rise as further reports are received. High-risk sexual behaviour is a major factor that has been linked to this rise. Indeed, behavioural surveillance data have demonstrated increases in rates of unprotected anal intercourse, and unprotected anal intercourse with HIV-positive or unknown status partners (Dodds and Mercey, 2003). Data from the second National Survey of Sexual Attitudes and Lifestyles suggest that there have been increases in the prevalence of male homosexual behaviour in the general population and increases in some high-risk behaviours among homosexually active men (Johnson *et al*, 2002). Continued liberalisation of attitudes towards homosexuality, and safer-sex fatigue in the era of antiretroviral therapy, coupled with expansions in sites that facilitate partner acquisition (eg. the internet, saunas) have been cited as possible contributing factors (Health Protection Agency, 2003a).

The HIV prevalence in injecting drug users attending specialist agencies is reported to have remained low, at less than 1%. In 2002, an estimated 1700 injecting drug users were living with HIV, and 300 of these were unaware of their infection. Of concern is the fact that over half of injecting drug users reported that they shared equipment in 2002 (Health Protection Agency, 2003a).

Since 1984, there have been five documented cases of occupationally-acquired HIV infections in healthcare workers in the UK, including one healthcare worker who seroconverted despite receiving post-exposure prophylaxis with triple therapy. Fourteen healthcare workers, with no risk factors other than an occupational exposure, have had HIV infections diagnosed in the UK. These were probably occupationally-acquired infections, although they do not have a baseline HIV negative test. All of these healthcare workers had worked in countries of higher HIV prevalence than the UK. For example, eleven of the fourteen had worked in sub-Saharan Africa (Health Protection Agency, 2003a).

In the UK, 1356 people have acquired HIV through blood product treatment. Some of these people received blood products in countries other than the UK. In addition, 372 people have become infected through being given a blood transfusion. Although, since 1985, viricidal heat treatment has routinely been performed, a few new cases of HIV infection attributed to receipt of blood transfusions have been reported. Almost all of these people have received transfusions in countries outside the UK where exclusion or screening procedures for donors are less rigorous. In the UK, four incidents of transfusion-associated transmission from two donors have occurred since screening began in 1985. Both donors were within the 'window period' between initial infection and the development of HIV antibodies (Health Protection Agency, 2003a).

By the end of 2002, a cumulative total of almost 56,000 diagnoses of HIV infection had been reported in the UK since the epidemic began in the early 1980s. Just over half of these people probably acquired their infection through homosexual sex. However, the distribution of HIV diagnoses across exposure categories has changed over the past ten years, with the rise in the number of new diagnoses in heterosexuals from 29% in 1993 to 57% in 2002. By the end of 2002, of the 1325 HIV diagnoses reported in children under fourteen years, 968 (73%) were reported to have acquired the infection from their mother. Most of the remainder were children infected with HIV through blood or blood product treatment. However, since the introduction of viral inactivation of blood products in 1985, there have been no reported transmissions by this route in the UK (Health Protection Agency, 2003a).

Other variations in the distribution of HIV and STIs in the general population have been reported. For example, high infection rates have been found among those with high rates of sexual partner change, particularly among homo/bisexual men and young heterosexuals. Geographic variations also exist, as can be seen in *Figures 1.9* and *1.10* (Health Protection Agency, 2003a).

The total number of infected people in the UK who accessed the Health Service for HIV-related care has risen by 20% since 2001, to 31,861 (*Figure 1.11*). This increase in care provision was particularly noticeable in areas bordering London. Both the rise in numbers of new diagnoses and the decrease in HIV-related deaths since the introduction of more effective therapies have contributed to this increase (Health Protection Agency, 2003a).

Homo/bisexual men remain the population sub-group with the greatest number of people seen for HIV-related care. Where ethnicity was reported among homo/bisexual men in 2002, the vast majority (88%) were white, 5% were mixed or other ethnicity, and 2% were Black-Caribbean.

The uptake of antiretroviral therapy is generally high, and there is no evidence that exposure category is associated with access to treatment (*Figure 1.12*).

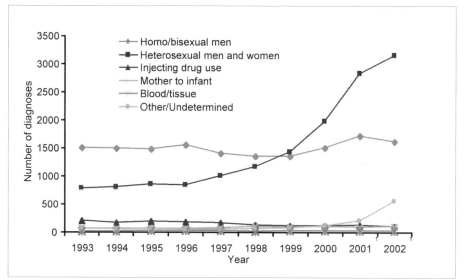

Figure 1.7: Exposure category of HIV-infected individuals by year of diagnosis in the UK, 1993–2002 (Health Protection Agency, 2003b). Numbers will rise for recent years, as further reports are received. Reported received by end of June 2003. Data source: HIV/AIDS report.

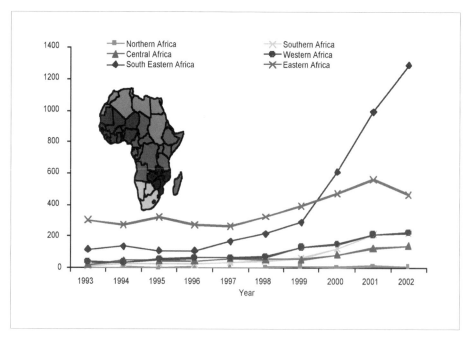

Figure 1.8: Probable region of infection[1] for heterosexual HIV infections that were probably acquired in Africa[2], 1993–2002 (Health Protection Agency, 2003b).

1   where the probable country of infection was a named country in Africa.
2   numbers will rise, for recent years, as further reports are received.

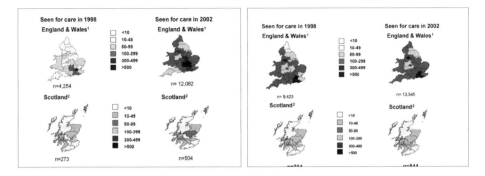

Figure 1.9: Numbers of diagnosed HIV-infected heterosexuals seen for care by residence[1], in England, Wales and Scotland, 1998 and 2002 (Health Protection Agency, 2003b)

1   Resident in England and Wales and for whom strategic Health Authority of residence was mapped.
2   Resident in Scotland and for whom NHS board of residence was mapped.

Data sources: SOPHID and CD4 Monitoring Scheme for Scotland.

Figure 1.10: Numbers of diagnosed HIV-infected homo/bisexual men seen for care by residence[1], in England, Wales and Scotland, 1998 and 2002 (Health Protection Agency, 2003b)

1   Resident in England and Wales and for whom strategic Health Authority of residence was mapped
2   Resident in Scotland and for whom NHS board of residence was mapped.

Data sources: SOPHID and CD4 Monitoring Scheme for Scotland.

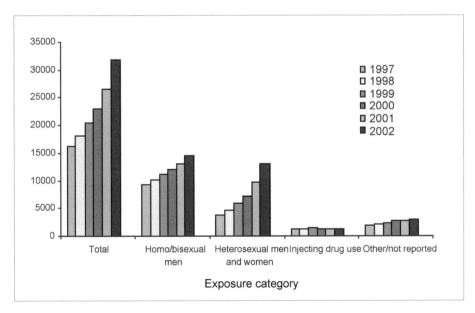

Figure 1.11: Diagnosed HIV-infected patients seen for care in the UK, 1997–2002 (Health Protection Agency, 2003b). Data sources: SOPHIC and CD4 Monitoring Scheme for Scotland.

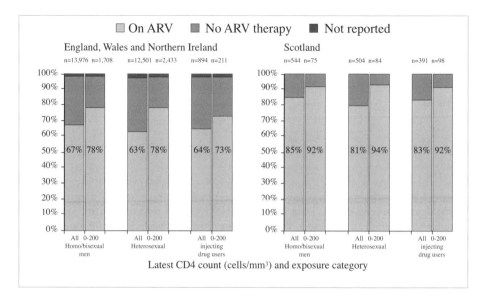

Figure 1.12: Proportion of HIV-infected patients on antiretroviral therapy (ARV) by exposure, category and clinical severity (Health Protection Agency, 2003b).
1   For Scotland, no ARV therapy includes patients for whom ARV therapy is not reported.
Data sources: SOPHID and CD4 Monitoring Scheme for Scotland.

Practice issues

Since 1997, combination antiretroviral therapy, preferably using three drugs including a protease inhibitor, has been effectively used to treat HIV infection (Randall, 1997). As referred to earlier, such treatment has resulted in an improved life expectancy. However, no cure for HIV has been found, and many under-privileged groups in industrialised countries have limited access to treatment. In addition, the social and economic situation in many developing countries restricts such treatment to the privileged few (Hankins, 1998). Prevention of HIV is therefore an important feature in relation to controlling the spread of HIV infection. Globally, people have been encouraged to abstain from sex and drugs, or insist that their partners use latex condoms (Shalala, 1996).

The challenges of preventing the spread of HIV are enormous. Globally, experts predict that most new infections will be among women, who are more vulnerable to infection for biological and socioeconomic reasons (Shalala, 1996). As the problem of HIV infection in the UK intensifies, policy makers are being urged to give urgent consideration to several key areas:

⌘ Reviewing and strengthening primary prevention efforts directed at homo/bisexual men.

⌘ Offering and recommending annual HIV testing to homo/bisexual men attending GUM clinics.

⌘ Promoting further voluntary confidential HIV testing of migrants from sub-Saharan Africa presenting at GUM clinics.

⌘ Developing further studies of the sexual behaviour of migrants from sub-Saharan Africa and HIV-infected people within the UK, in order to better inform primary and secondary prevention efforts.

⌘ Devoting increased resources to risk factor follow-up of newly diagnosed HIV-infected heterosexuals.

⌘ Reducing the current length of waiting times to GUM clinics.

(Health Protection Agency, 2003)

In addition, because young people bear a disproportionate burden of acute STIs (Health Protection Agency, 2003), The English National Strategy for Sexual Health and HIV (DoH, 2002) has specifically identified young people as a priority group for interventions and research. Interventions that have been implemented include sex and relationship education in schools, health promotion through the 'Sex Lottery Campaign', one-stop shops and youth-friendly services. Effective secondary services are essential in tackling the growing problem of secondary re-infection (Health Protection Agency, 2003).

Midwives are expected to contribute to the development and evaluation of guidelines and policies and make recommendations for change in the interests of women, babies and their families. In addition, they are required to contribute to enhancing the health and social wellbeing of individuals and their communities, and to support the creation and maintenance of environments that promote the health, safety and wellbeing of women, babies and others (NMC, 2004). The Safer Sex Enterprise is an example of a recent initiative that was set up in Wales to enable young people to have easier access to sexual health advice and contraception. Midwives work alongside youth workers, undertaking the following activities:

• distributing leaflets and condoms to teenagers on the streets of targeted towns
• providing group sessions on 'sex education'
• providing confidential one-to-one information
• offering pregnancy testing.

Initial evaluation of qualitative data suggests that the service is both popular with young people and effective in providing them with sexual health advice (Lewis, 2004).

In practice, midwives should be able to improve awareness of HIV among women and their families, and encourage women to adopt healthy or safer patterns of sexual behaviour. In addition, midwives are required to offer and recommend HIV screening during pregnancy (DoH, 1999). Improving diagnosis rates will enable infected women to make informed choices regarding interventions to reduce the risk of mother-to-child transmission of HIV infection from 25%–30% to less than 2% (Low-Beer and Smith, 2004). Services for pregnant women and their families should be sensitive to the special needs of particular groups, such as teenagers and communities from sub-Saharan Africa. Meanwhile, the hunt for a vaccine is ongoing (WHO, 2004).

Conclusion

HIV infection is a continuing problem as the global and national spread of the disease appears to be unhalted. Prevention of infection continues to be an important challenge, although from a global perspective, socioeconomic factors influence the effectiveness of health education among women, who are more vulnerable to infection than men. In addition to offering and recommending screening for HIV during pregnancy, midwives have a key role in sexual health promotion. The special needs of young women and teenagers, and women from ethnic minority groups, are particularly challenging.

References

Adler WM, ed (1997) *ABC of AIDS*. 4th edn. BMJ Books, London

Department of Health (1999) *Targets aimed at reducing the number of children born with HIV: report from an expert group*. DoH, London

Department of Health (2002) *The National Strategy for Sexual Health and HIV implementation action plan*. DoH, London

Dodds J, Mercey D (2003) *Sexual health survey of gay men — London 2002: summary of results*. Royal Free and University College Medical School, London

Hankins C (1998) 12th World AIDS Conference. Epidemiology, Prevention and Public Health Track C (online). Available online: http://www.aids98. ch/archive/1_WEDNESDAY/010798_summarysession_trackc.html (accessed 24 June, 2004)

Health Protection Agency, SCIEH, ISD, National Public Health Service for Wales, CDSC Northern Ireland and the UASSG (2003a) *Renewing the focus. HIV and other Sexually Transmitted Infections in the United Kingdom in 2002*. Health Protection Agency, London

Health Protection Agency (2003b) *Renewing the focus. HIV and other Sexually Transmitted Infections in the United Kingdom in 2002*. Core Slides, November 2003 (online). Available online: http://www.hpa.org.uk/ infections/topics_az/hiv_and_sti/publications/annual2003/annual2003.htm

Heaphy S (1999) *Virus Structure* (online). Available online: http://www.tulane. edu/~dmsander/WWW/335/335Structure.html (accessed 15 June, 2004)

Ho DD (1996) Viral counts count in HIV infection. *Science* **272**: 1124–25. Available online: http://www.images.md/users/explore–collection.asp (accessed 21 October, 2004)

Johnson AM, Dodds J, Mercer CH, Fenton KA, Wellings K, Erens B *et al* (2002) HIV changing patterns of male homosexual behaviour in Britain: comparative analysis of independent community and national probability samples (Natsal) 1990–2001. Oral presentation at IUSTI-Europe 2002 18th Congress on Sexually Transmitted Infections. Vienna, 12–14

Lewis M (2004) Working together to make a difference. *Midwives* **7**(10): 422–3

Low-Beer NM, Smith JR (2004) *Management of HIV in Pregnancy*. RCOG Guideline No. 39. Royal College of Obstetricians and Gynaecologists (online). Available online: http://www.rcog.org.uk/guidelines (accessed 30th June 2004)

Nursing and Midwifery Council (2004) *Standards of Proficiency for pre-registration midwifery education*. NMC, London

Perez K, Saag M, Kilby J (2001) *Atlas of Infectious Diseases: AIDS*. Current Medicine LLC. Available online: http://www.images.md/users/explore_collection.asp (accessed 21 October, 2004)

Pratt R (1995) *HIV and AIDS. A Strategy for Nursing Care*. 4th edn, Edward Arnold, London

Randall P (1997) Draft HIV/AIDS Treatment Guidelines Available (online). Available online: http://www.niaid.nih.gov/newsroom/guidelines.htm (accessed 24 June, 2004)

Shalala DE (1996) Plenary Address, 11th International Conference on AIDS (online). Available online: http://www.os.dhhs.gov/news/speeches/vanplen.html (accessed 28 June, 2004)

School of Medical Sciences, Otago University (1998) Human Immunodeficiency Virus (HIV) (online). Available online: http://osms.otago.ac.nz/bur_AIDS.htm (accessed 24 June, 2004)

Toebe C (1999) HIV origins, subtypes and viral replication (online). Available online: http://cloud.ccsf.cc.ca.us/Departments/Biology/HIVtypes.htm#What is a Retrovirus?? (accessed 15 June, 2004)

UNAIDS (2004a) Questions & Answers II: Basic facts about the HIV/AIDS epidemic and its impact (online). Available online: http://www.unaids.org/EN/other/functionalities/Search.asp (accessed 15 October, 2004)

UNAIDS (2004b) 2004 Report on the global AIDS epidemic. Executive Summary (online). Available online: http://www.unaids.org/en/default.asp (accessed 25 October, 2004)

World Health Organization (2004) HIV vaccine trial results are an important step forward in developing an effective vaccine, say WHO and UNAIDS (online). Available online: http://www.who.int/mediacentre/releases/2003/pr19/en/ (accessed 30 June, 2004)

Chapter 2

HIV and women: health and childbearing issues

This chapter will examine the effect of HIV on women's health, and will include discussion of gender differences related to disease progression, the use of antiretroviral therapy, and sexual and reproductive issues. Women with known HIV infection may previously have avoided pregnancy because of their serostatus. Now, with the promise of new therapies that both improve their own health and longevity and reduce the risk of vertical transmission, they are reconsidering their reproductive options (Beckerman, 1998). In addition, more women are choosing to take up the offer of HIV testing during pregnancy (Health Protection Agency, 2003), and therefore the number of women diagnosed will increase. An understanding of HIV-related health and childbearing issues will enable midwives to help women make informed decisions before they conceive and during pregnancy.

Therapeutic recommendations regarding HIV disease have changed at a rate that far outpaces the appearance of published texts, and the best resource for learning the latest findings about HIV is by direct consultation with experts or from constantly updated websites (Beckerman, 1998).

Heterosexual transmission

Heterosexual intercourse is the primary mode of HIV infection worldwide. Recommendations for the prevention of sexually transmitted HIV include abstinence, long-term monogamy with a sero-negative partner, or a limited number of lifetime sexual partners. The use of condoms is recommended for each and every act of intercourse where people have multiple partners, or a primary partner who is infected, or whose partner's serostatus is unknown (CDC, 1988; Surgeon General, 1993; CDC, 1993). Consistent use of condoms has been associated with an 80% reduction in HIV transmission (Weller and Davis, 2002).

Women are eight times more likely to become infected through heterosexual transmission of HIV than men (Newman, 1998). Other factors that increase the risk still further include the presence of sexually transmitted infections (STIs) and genital ulcers, an increased number of sexual contacts, the use of intra-uterine contraceptive devices (IUCDs), an advanced state of HIV disease progression in the partner, and participation in anal sex (Newman, 1998).

Uninfected women wishing to conceive with an HIV-infected partner would expose themselves to an estimated risk of transmission of 1:500 per sexual act (Mandelbrot, 1997). This risk may be reduced by restricting intercourse to the time surrounding ovulation. A safer option involves semen-washing coupled with reproductive technology to eliminate the risk of transmission. Semen-washing reduces both HIV RNA and DNA to undetectable amounts (Semprini and Fiore, 2004). Indeed, there have been no seroconversions in women inseminated with washed sperm, and this service is now available in a number of centres across the UK (Low-Beer and Smith, 2004). Semen-washing may also be offered when both partners are infected with different viral strains (Semprini and Fiore, 2004).

HIV-infected women wishing to conceive with an uninfected partner can perform artificial insemination around the time of ovulation (Low-Beer and Smith, 2004).

HIV in lesbians

Although the number of documented women-to-women transmissions is low (Newman, 1998), women partners of HIV-infected women should be advised to avoid mucus membrane contact of all potentially infectious secretions (Norman *et al*, 1996; White, 1997).

Gender differences and disease progression

Initial studies suggested that there was a difference in disease progression and survival between men and women. However, more recent studies have indicated that these earlier studies were related more to poor access to medical care for women than to gender differences (Newman, 1998).

Age at the time of infection with HIV is a more important determinant of survival, as is shown by the findings of a study involving 1216 HIV-infected haemophiliacs in the UK (*Figure 2.1*). Overall, 67% of the study population were still living ten years after sero-conversion, with the younger age groups surviving even longer. The apparent steep age gradient in survival was not explained by deaths expected in the absence of HIV infection or by other confounding factors such as haemophilia severity or type (Darby *et al*, 1996).

Symptoms of middle-stage HIV disease in women are non-specific and similar to those in men, for example, night sweats, fatigue, diarrhoea, weight loss and a cough (Carpenter *et al*, 1991; Hankins and Handley, 1992). Generally, no obvious differences between the sexes have been found in the presentation and natural history of common AIDS-defining illnesses such as *Pneumocystis carinii* pneumonia and toxoplasmosis (Newman, 1998). However, Karposi's sarcoma, a malignant condition occurring frequently in HIV-infected homosexual men, occurs in less than 2% of HIV-infected women. Women who develop Karposi's sarcoma are more likely to have had sex with a bisexual man, although it has occurred in women who became infected with HIV through injecting drug use or blood transfusion (Newman, 1998). Unusual presentations of Karposi's sarcoma in women have been reported, for example, vulva pain, vaginal discharge and a vulval mass (Macasaet *et al*, 1995).

Most HIV-infected homosexual men have a positive IgG antibody test for cytomegalovirus (CMV). However, rates in women are similar to those in the general population, in which 50% of adults are sero-positive (Newman, 1998). Care should be taken to ensure that pregnant women are tested for CMV antibodies, and CMV-negative women who require a blood transfusion during childbirth should always be given CMV-negative blood to avoid future risk of CMV end-organ disease.

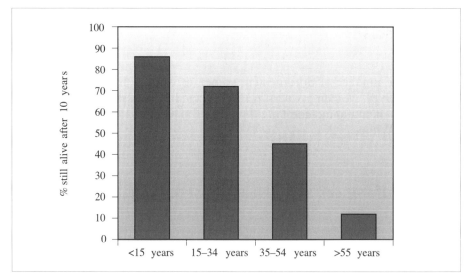

Figure 2.1: Findings of a study involving 1216 HIV-infected haemophiliacs in the UK

Gynaecological disease

HIV-infected women, particularly those with advanced immunosuppression, may experience various gynaecological disorders that may be more frequent, more severe and less responsive to therapy, compared with uninfected women (Newman, 2004).

Vaginal infections

Vaginal candidiasis, a frequent disorder in the general population, can cause morbidity in HIV-infected women. Although this condition may affect women in early or late HIV disease, many women with severe immunosuppression do not become infected (Newman, 1998). Other vaginal infections, which may occur more frequently in HIV-infected women, include trichomoniasis, bacterial vaginosis, syphilis, gonorrhea and chlamydia (Anastos *et al*, 1997).

Genital warts

HIV-infected women are more prone to recurrence of genital warts, compared with non-HIV infected women (Newman, 1998). One study has reported a ten-fold increase in genital warts (Greenblatt *et al*, 1996).

Genital herpes

Herpes simplex virus, which affects women in the general population, may also affect HIV-infected women, in the form of severe ulcerative genital herpes, which is an AIDS-defining illness (Carpenter *et al*, 1991). Common sites of presentation of herpes simplex virus, which recurs more frequently in HIV-infected women, include the labia majora and minora, the sacrum and the buttocks (Newman, 1998).

Genital ulcerative disease

Herpes simplex virus, cytomegalovirus (CMV), syphilis, gonorrhoea, other bacterial or fungal pathogens, and malignancies may cause genital ulcerative disease, which is painful and difficult to treat (Newman, 1998).

Pelvic inflammatory disease

Pelvic inflammatory disease may be more severe in women with advanced HIV disease. For example, 25% of HIV-infected women with this disease developed a tubo-ovarian abscess, compared with only 12% of non-HIV infected women in a control group (Newman, 1998).

Cervical cytological abnormalities

HIV-infected women have an increased incidence and aggressiveness of cervical cancer, compared with non-HIV infected women (Newman, 1998). Women in more advanced stages of immunosuppression tend to have more advanced cervical intraepithelial neoplasia (Newman, 2004). Human papilloma virus (HPV) is an aetiological factor in cervical cancer, and HIV-related immunosuppression makes women particularly susceptible to HPV infection.

As cervical intraepithelial neoplasia is more frequent and more aggressive in women with severe immunosuppression, some authorities recommend performing a Pap smear every six months for women with more advanced immunodeficiency (Minkoff and DeHovitz, 1991; Anastos *et al*, 1997; Newman, 1998). Indeed, Newman (2004) recommends six-monthly smears in addition to careful vulva, vaginal and anal inspection, especially in patients with CD4 counts of less than 200 cells/μL. However, clinical guidelines should be modified for individual patients as appropriate — for example, in cases where a woman has previously had a negative smear result and is currently in the final stage of disease progression (Anastos *et al*, 1997), or during pregnancy, as pregnancy does not affect the incidence of abnormal smears (Stratton *et al*, 1996).

Anal squamous intraepithelial neoplasia

Anal squamous intraepithelial neoplasia is also more prevalent among HIV-infected women (Melbye *et al*, 1993). As with cervical intraepithelial neoplasia, the likelihood of cytological abnormalities is greater in women who are more immunosuppressed (Newman, 1998).

Antiretroviral treatment

For women of reproductive age, the indications for initiation of antiretroviral therapy and the goals of treatment are the same as for other adults and adolescents (Panel on Clinical Practices for Treatment of HIV Infection convened by the Department of Health and Human Services [DHHS], 2004). Studies suggest that current combinations of antiretroviral therapy are as equally effective in women as in men (Newman, 1998). Early initiation of aggressive combination antiretroviral regimes to suppress maximally viral replication, preserve immune function and reduce the development of resistance, is recommended (Havlir and Richman, 1996). The new, potent antiretroviral drugs that inhibit the protease enzyme of HIV-1, when used in combination with nucleoside analogue reverse transcriptase inhibitors, reduce plasma HIV-1 RNA levels for prolonged periods to levels that are undetectable with current assays. This has resulted in improved clinical outcome and survival in adults receiving such regimens (Hammer *et al*, 1997; Gulick *et al*, 1997).

Given that they have a lower mean body weight, and lower mean haemoglobin levels compared with men, women may be more susceptible to the toxic effects of antiretroviral therapy, including anaemia (Newman, 1998). Side-effects of antiretroviral therapy are similar in both men and women. However, nausea and vomiting may be particularly problematic for women during pregnancy. Other reported side-effects include malaise, fatigue, perioral numbness and tingling, diarrhoea, abdominal pain, itching and skin rash (Currier *et al*, 1997; Gersten *et al*, 1997; Ocamb *et al*, 1997).

It is important that women strictly adhere to their medication regimens to prevent the development of drug resistance. In addition, when planning treatment, the possibility of planned or unplanned pregnancy should be considered. The most vulnerable period in fetal organogenesis is during the first few weeks of gestation, when the woman may not be aware she is pregnant. Women should be informed about the potential teratogenic risk of efavirenz-containing regimens should pregnancy occur. These regimens should be avoided in women who are trying to conceive or who are not using effective and consistent contraception. It is important that sexual activity, reproductive plans and use of effective contraception are discussed with women (Panel on Clinical Practices for Treatment of HIV Infection convened by the Department of Health and Human Services [DHHS], 2004).

Several studies have found that women have lower viral loads than men have at a similar CD4 cell count (Gandhi *et al*, 2002). These differences in viral load occur predominantly during the phase of the illness when the CD4 cell count is relatively preserved. Doctors may consider lower plasma HIV RNA thresholds for initiating antiretroviral therapy in women with CD4 cell counts exceeding 350 cells/mm^3, although an appropriate threshold has not been determined (Newman, 2004). Given that only very small sex-based differences in viral load are apparent in patients with CD4 cell counts of less than 350 cells/mm^3, no changes in treatment guidelines for women are recommended (DHHS and the Henry J Kaiser Family Foundation, 2003).

Sexual and reproductive issues

Many women experience temporary 'loss of libido' when they are initially given an HIV diagnosis (Anastos *et al*, 1997). If this is a problem following routine antenatal screening, midwives should reassure women that sexual interest will resume.

Reproductive counselling for HIV-infected women should be educational, supportive and non-directive (Beckerman, 1998). HIV-infected women have a right to make choices in relation to childbearing, and they should be given relevant information to enable them to exercise that right. Reproductive choices and options should be discussed in a sensitive and non-judgmental way. *In-vitro* fertilisation (IVF) is now considered ethically acceptable for couples seeking assisted reproduction, since vertical transmission rates are now greatly reduced and life expectancy for parents taking HAART (highly active antiretroviral therapy) is increased (Low-Beer and Smith, 2004; Gilling-Smith *et al*, 2001).

Varying rates of vertical transmission have been reported, ranging from 15%–20% in Europe, 15%–30% in the USA and 23%–35% in Africa (Newell and Peckham, 1993). In addition, babies can become infected with HIV as a result of breast-feeding, which adds another 7%–22% to the risk of transmission (Dunn, 1992). The risk may be reduced to below 2% by giving antiretroviral therapy to the mother and baby, performing an elective caesarean section and avoiding breast-feeding (European Collaborative Study, 2001). HIV-infected women would need to consider the possible embryonic or fetal toxicity associated with antiretroviral therapy and, although caesarean section has a proven protective efficacy without significant maternal morbidity, its role is now being re-evaluated in mothers with undetectable viral load.

Breast-feeding, discouraged to avoid postnatal transmission, might be possible in the future when antiretroviral therapy capable of suppressing viral excretion in maternal milk is developed (Semprini and Fiore, 2004). In the meantime, however, the Department of Health has issued updated guidance following a review of the research evidence, reaffirming existing advice. Midwives should continue to advise HIV-infected women and new mothers, recommending the avoidance of breast-feeding as part of a programme of interventions to reduce the risk of mother-to-child HIV transmission (UK Chief Medical Officers' Expert Advisory Group on AIDS, 2004).

Practical support for women to bottle feed may involve assisting them to overcome social and cultural barriers. For example, in cultures where breast-feeding is the norm, HIV-infected mothers may feel that bottle feeding highlights the possibility of infection. Fear of violence, stigma, ostracism or being abandoned if their HIV-status were exposed may make it difficult for them to avoid breast-feeding (UK Chief Medical Officers' Expert Advisory Group on AIDS, 2004). Voluntary organisations can provide in-valuable sources of further support and advice for women and their families affected by HIV. Midwives should be able to give women relevant information and telephone helpline numbers (*Table 2.1*). When bottle-feeding is not the norm, midwives should ensure women are given appropriate advice and support to

Table 2.1: Voluntary organisations and helplines	
African AIDS helpline	0800 0965 500
Positively women	0208 7713 0222
Terence Higgins Trust	0845 1221 200
Ugandan AIDS Action fund	020 7928 9583

bottle feed their babies safely. Women from disadvantaged groups may require help to access financial assistance from social services. For example, pregnant asylum seekers, who are in receipt of support from the National Asylum Support Service (NASS) are eligible to receive additional cash payments for themselves and dependant children under the age of three (NASS Policy Bulletin 78, 2004). These benefits are similar to that of milk tokens under the Welfare Food Scheme, and may be used to buy bottle feeds.

When HIV-infected mothers choose to breast-feed, midwives should be aware that under the Children Act 1989, courts have a statutory duty to treat the welfare of the baby as paramount. The Act places a general duty on every local authority to safeguard and promote the welfare of children within their area who are in need (UK Chief Medical Officers' Expert Advisory Group on AIDS, 2004). Midwives may find themselves in a difficult position, as their duty of care to the mother may conflict with the needs of the baby. It is vital to ensure (by use of an interpreter, for example) if there are language difficulties, that the mother understands why bottle-feeding is recommended and to explore the reasons why a mother might feel unable to avoid breast-feeding.

In exceptional circumstances, the midwife may be required to support an HIV-infected mother who persists in wanting to breast-feed her baby. The midwife should ensure that she informs the social worker, the paediatrician and her supervisor of midwives. Accurate and factual records of all care and advice should be kept. To protect the infant from possible transmission of HIV infection through breastfeeding, the DoH guidance for healthcare professionals suggests several strategies that would minimise the risk (UK Chief Medical Officers' Expert Advisory Group on AIDS, 2004). A midwife who finds herself in the difficult position of supporting an HIV-infected mother who chooses to breast-feed her baby should advise the mother of these strategies:

- antiretroviral drug therapy for the mother and her baby
- exclusive breast-feeding, ie. avoid infant formula milk supplements or other fluids
- early discontinuation of breast-feeding, substituting infant formula milk for breast milk before six months or solid foods after six months
- ensuring correct positioning and attachment of the baby to the breast.

Midwives should provide advice, support and help to enable the mother to attach her baby to the breast correctly, especially for the first few feeds. The aim of care is to prevent cracked nipples and mastitis, which may increase the risk of mother-to-child transmission of HIV (Pillay *et al*, 2000). Midwives should also examine the baby's mouth to detect signs of oral candidiasis, which should be treated promptly, as this may also increase the risk of transmission. Recurrent severe candidiasis can be a sign of HIV infection in the baby (UK Chief Medical Officers' Expert Advisory Group on AIDS, 2004).

Contraceptive choices should also be discussed, including knowledge of the particular advantages and disadvantages of different methods of contraception, so that women can make an informed choice after the birth of their baby. Relevant information from the available literature (Anastos *et al*, 1997; (Newman, 1998) has been summarised in *Table 2.2*.

Table 2.2: Contraceptive choices and HIV
Male condoms with spermicides
❖ Excellent choice when acceptable to both partners ❖ Possible allergic reaction
Female condom
❖ Enables women to be in control if its used. This is an issue for many women who may be unable to negotiate 'safer sex' in terms of male condom use ❖ The polyurethane sheath partially covers the external vagina, providing protection against HIV, cytomegalovirus and hepatitis B ❖ Has the same contraceptive efficacy as other barrier methods, including the male condom
Diaphragm with spermicide
❖ Good contraceptive choice ❖ Does not prevent (although it may limit) transmission of STDs
Intra-uterine contraceptive devices
❖ Carries a high risk of infection, and therefore not a good choice for immunocompromised women ❖ The 'Mirena' IUCD may be an acceptable choice for women at low risk for STIs
Oral contraceptives
❖ Some drugs used in the treatment of HIV, such as ritonavir or nelfinavir (protease inhibitors) and nevirapine (a non-nucleoside reverse transcriptase inhibitor), may substantially reduce the bioavailability of ethinyl estradiol ❖ A potential increased risk of gingivitis, respiratory infections and vaginitis ❖ A possible reduced immune function in immunocompromised women ❖ Theoretical decreased risk of pelvic inflammatory disease
Depo-provera (intramuscular progesterone)
❖ An efficient contraceptive which lasts for three months ❖ Can cause irregular bleeding ❖ Uncertain hormonal interaction in HIV illness ❖ Uncertain interactions with drugs commonly used in HIV
Norplant (progesterone implants)
❖ An efficient contraceptive which lasts for five years ❖ Can cause irregular bleeding ❖ Uncertain hormonal interaction in HIV illness ❖ Increased risk of infection at site of insertion in immunocompromised women ❖ Uncertain interactions with drugs commonly used in HIV
Sterilisation
❖ Excellent permanent method of contraception ❖ Does not prevent transmission of STIs

The intrauterine contraceptive device was relatively contraindicated in the past because of concerns regarding its associated risk of pelvic inflammatory disease.

However, the 'Mirena' device, in particular, may be an acceptable alternative for women with a low risk of STIs. Women should be informed of its association with pelvic inflammatory disease, and periodic screening for *Neisseria gonorrhoea* and *Chlamydia trachomatis* should be considered (Watts, 2002).

Effects of pregnancy on HIV progression

There is no evidence of an association between adverse maternal outcomes and pregnancy in HIV-infected women. However, further larger studies need to be done before this issue can be resolved (French and Brocklehurst, 1998a).

HIV and pregnancy outcomes

French and Brocklehurst (1998b) undertook a systematic review of the literature and meta-analysis, and found an association between maternal HIV infection and an adverse perinatal outcome. The risk of spontaneous abortion was 2.8–6 times higher in HIV-infected women compared with non-infected women, and there was a greatly increased risk of infant death in developing countries. No association was found in relation to fetal abnormalities.

Other researchers have concluded that HIV-infected women, particularly those who are symptomatic, have a higher risk of adverse pregnancy outcomes (Coley *et al*, 2001). In Tanzania, 1078 HIV-infected and 502 uninfected women between twelve and twenty-seven weeks of gestation were studied. After controlling for potential confounding factors, the researchers found no significant differences between uninfected women and HIV-infected women in their risks of fetal loss, low birth weight or weight, head circumference and gestational age of the babies at birth. However, HIV-infected women were more likely to deliver severely premature babies (<34 weeks). Also, there was a significantly higher risk of low birth weight and prematurity (<37 weeks) among symptomatic HIV-infected women when compared with uninfected women.

The effects of antiretroviral therapy on pregnancy outcomes have also been studied. One study involved 2123 HIV-1-infected pregnant women who were treated as follows:

- 1590 were given monotherapy
- 396 were given combination therapy without protease inhibitors
- 137 were given combination therapy with protease inhibitors
- 1143 women did not receive antiretroviral therapy.

The findings showed a similar rate of premature delivery among the women who received antiretroviral therapy and those who did not (16% and 17%, respectively) after adjustment for multiple risk factors, including the CD4 cell count and use or non-use of tobacco, alcohol and illicit drugs. The rate of low birth weight (<2500g) was 16% in both groups, and the rate of very low birth weight (<1500g) was 2% among the group that received antiretroviral therapy and 1% in the group that did not. The rates of low Apgar scores (<7) and stillbirth were also similar or the same in the two groups.

Compared with monotherapy, combination antiretroviral therapy was not associated with an increased risk of premature delivery or delivery of a low birth weight baby. Seven of the women who received combination therapy with protease inhibitors (5%) had babies whose birth weights were very low, as compared with nine women who received combination therapy without protease inhibitors (2%).

The researchers concluded that combination therapy, compared with no antiretroviral therapy or monotherapy, is not associated with increased rates of premature delivery, low birth weight, low Apgar scores, or stillbirth. However, the association between combination therapy with protease inhibitors and an increased risk of very low birth weight requires confirmation (Tuomala *et al*, 2002). In addition, the report from the European Collaborative Study found no difference in the rate of birth defects among 906 infants (rate 1.4%) compared with 1508 infants (rate 1.6%) without antiretroviral exposure during pregnancy (European Collaborative Study, 2003).

Increasing numbers of women entering pregnancy on multiple antiretroviral agents are being referred to the Antiretroviral Pregnancy Registry (APR), which monitors prenatal exposures to antiretroviral drugs and pregnancy outcome. Since the APR started receiving reports in 1989, through to July 2003, 3583 live births have been monitored. The data show no increase in prevalence of birth defects overall among women exposed to lamivudine, nelfinavir, nevirapine, stavudine, and zidovudine (Watts *et al*, 2004).

The challenges facing midwives are enormously wide-ranging and complex. Midwives are required to be responsive to individualised needs, well-informed, and continuously educated in relation to the latest research and DoH guidelines for good practice. To assist healthcare professionals working in maternity care, the Royal College of Midwives (RCM) and the DoH have published recommendations for developing effective services (*Table 2.3*).

Conclusion

A developing knowledge-base and advances in the management of HIV have resulted in fresh hope for many women who are given an HIV diagnosis. With appropriate interventions, particularly the use of newer antiretroviral therapies both during and after pregnancy, many HIV-infected women in the developed world will not only be able to anticipate that their babies will be born uninfected, but also that they themselves will have a significant chance of living long enough to see their children grow to adulthood (Beckerman, 1998). HIV poses enormous challenges for midwives. Midwives should face these challenges and consider adopting the practice recommendations laid out by the RCM and DoH, so that effective and supportive services are provided for affected women and their babies.

Table 2.3: Practice recommendations for midwives in HIV and maternity care
❖ All maternity units should develop multidisciplinary protocols on all aspects of HIV testing and the care of women who are infected with HIV
❖ All midwives need to be aware of, and understand, the Children Act, the child protection policies of their local authority, and their own statutory responsibilities in relation to child protection
❖ Managers and supervisors of midwives should ensure that all midwives fully understand their role and responsibilities in relation to HIV issues, including antenatal testing and infant feeding
❖ Midwives should develop local strategies to facilitate informed choice on infant feeding
❖ HIV-infected women who feel strongly committed to breast-feeding should be assisted to explore ways to reduce the risk of doing so
❖ Maternity services should monitor and audit the implementation of policies and protocols around HIV infection and infant feeding, to ensure their effectiveness and acceptability for both users and staff
❖ Midwives who are concerned that local policy or practice conflicts with their professional and ethical responsibilities, or with women's best interests, should consult their supervisor of midwives or the RCM
❖ Midwives should actively promote best practice in this area by sharing their experiences and expertise with others
❖ Midwives should strive to offer services that are sensitive, culturally appropriate, accessible and trusted by women with HIV infection
❖ Care should be taken to ensure that supporting HIV-infected women to give infant formula milk does not undermine the promotion of breast-feeding, which remains the best way to feed the majority of infants in the UK

References

Anastos K, Denenberg R, Solomon L (1997) Human immunodeficiency virus infection in women. *Med Clin North Am* **81**(2): 533–53

Beckerman KP (1998) Reproduction and HIV disease: Pregnancy and perinatal care of HIV-1-infected women. In: Cohen PT, ed. *Natural History, Clinical Spectrum, and General Management of HIV Disease* (online). Available online: http://hivinsite.ucsf.edu/akb/1997/04preg/index. html (accessed 12th August 1999)

Carpenter CC, Mayer KH, Stein MD, Leibman BD, Fisher A, Fiore TC (1991) Human immunodeficiency virus infection in North American women: experience with 200 cases and a review of the literature. *Medicine* (Baltimore) **70**(5): 307–25

Centers for Disease Control (1988) Condoms for prevention of sexually transmitted diseases. *MMWR* **37**: 133–7

Centers for Disease Control (1993) Update: Barrier protection against HIV infection and other sexually transmitted diseases. *MMWR* **42**: 589–591, 597

Coley JL, Msamanga GI, Smith Fawzi MC, Kaaya S, Hertzmark E, Kapiga S *et al* (2001) The association between maternal HIV-1 infection and pregnancy outcomes in Dar es Salaam, Tanzania. *Br J Obstet Gynaecol* **108**(11): 1125–33

Currier JS, Yetzer E, Potthoff A, Glassman H, Heath-Chiozzi M (1997) Gender differences in adverse events on ritonavir: an analysis from the Abbott 247 study. In: Proceedings of the National Conference on Women and HIV, Pasadena: 154 (abstract no 304.7)

Darby SC, Ewart DW, Giangrande PL, Spooner RJ, Rizza CR (1996) Importance of age at infection with HIV-1 for survival and development of AIDS in UK haemophilia population. *Lancet* **347**(9015):1573–9

DHHS and the Henry J Kaiser Family Foundation (2003) *Guidelines for the Use of Antiretroviral Agents in HIV-1-Infected Adults and Adolescents.* Supplement: Considerations for Antiretroviral Therapy in Women. Available online: http://aidsinfo.nih.gov/guidelines/adult/CW_111003.html

Dunn DT, Newell ML, Aden AE *et al* (1992) Risk of human immunodeficiency virus type 1 transmission through breast-feeding. *Lancet* **340**: 585–8

European Collaborative Study (2001) HIV-infected pregnant women and vertical transmission in Europe since 1986. *J AIDS* **15**: 761–70

European Collaborative Study (2003) Exposure to antiretroviral therapy in utero or early life: the health of uninfected children born to HIV-infected women. *J AIDS* **32**: 380–7

French R, Brocklehurst P (1998a) The effect of pregnancy on survival in women infected with HIV: a systematic review of the literature and meta-analysis. *Br J Obstet Gynaecol* **105**(8): 827–35

French R, Brocklehurst P (1998b) The association between maternal HIV infection and perinatal outcome: a systematic review of the literature and meta-analysis. *Br J Obstet Gynaecol* **105**(8): 836–48

Gandhi M, Bacchetti P, Miotti P, Quinn TC, Veronese F, Greenblatt RM (2002) Does patient sex affect human immunodeficiency virus levels? *Clin Infect Dis* **35**(3): 313–22

Gersten M, Chapman S, Farnsworth A, Chang Y, Yu G, Clendeninn N (1997) *The safety and efficacy of Viracept (nelfinavir mesylate, NFV) in female patients who participated in pivotal phase II/III double-blind randomized controlled trials*. In: Proceedings of the National Conference on Women and HIV, Pasadena: 152 (abstract no 304.1)

Gilling-Smith C, Smith JR, Semprini AE (2001) HIV and infertility: time to treat. There's no justification for denying treatment to parents who are HIV positive. *Br Med J* **322**: 566–7

Greenblatt RM, Barkan S, Delepena R *et al* and the Women's Interagency HIV Study (1996) *Lower genital tract infections among HIV infected women and high seronegatives: The Women's Interagency HIV Study*. 11th World AIDS Conference

Gulick RM, Mellors JW, Havlir D *et al* (1997) Treatment with indinavir, zidovudine and lamivudine in adults with human immunodeficiency virus infection and prior antiretroviral therapy. *N Engl J Med* **337**: 734–9

Hammer SM, Squires KE, Hughes MD *et al* (1997) A controlled trial of two nucleoside analogues plus indinavir in persons with human immunodeficiency virus infection and CD4 cell counts of 200 per cubic millimeter or less. *N Engl J Med* **337**: 725–33

Hankins CA, Handley MA (1992) HIV disease and AIDS in women: current knowledge and a research agenda. *J Acquir Immune Defic Syndr* (10): 957–71

Havlir DV, Richman DD (1996) Viral dynamics of HIV: implications for drug development and therapeutic strategies. *Ann Intern Med* **124**: 984–94

Health Protection Agency, SCIEH, ISD, National Public Health Service for Wales, CDSC Northern Ireland and the UASSG (2003) *Renewing the focus. HIV and other Sexually Transmitted Infections in the United Kingdom in 2002*. Health Protection Agency, London

Low-Beer NM, Smith JR (2004) Management of HIV in Pregnancy. RCOG Guideline No 39, Royal College of Obstetricians and Gynaecologists (online). Available online: http://www.rcog.org.uk/guidelines (accessed 30th June 2004)

Macasaet MA, Duerr A, Thelmo W, Vernon SD, Unger ER (1995) Kaposi sarcoma presenting as a vulvar mass. *Obstet Gynecol* **86**: 695–7

Mandelbrot L, Heard I, Henrion-Geant E, Henrion R (1997) Natural conception in HIV-negative women with HIV-infected partners. *Lancet* **349**: 850–1

Melbye M, Cote T, Biggar RJ, Rabkin C (1993) High incidence of anal cancer among AIDS patients — a merge analysis of AIDS and cancer registries in the USA. *Int Conf AIDS* **9**(1): 408 (abstract no. PO-B14-1636)

Minkoff HL, DeHovitz JA (1991) Care of women infected with the human immunodeficiency virus. *JAMA.* **266**(16): 2253–8

Nass Bulletin 78 (2004) *Additional payments to pregnant women and children aged under 3* (online). Available online: http://www.ind.homeoffice. gov.uk/ind/en/home/applying/national_asylum_support/policy_bulletin/ additional_payments.html? (accessed 4 November, 2004)

Newell ML, Peckham C (1993) Risk factors for vertical transmission of HIV-1 and early markers of HIV-1 infection in children. *AIDS* **7**(suppl 1): S91–97)

Newman (1998) Women and HIV disease. In: Cohen PT, ed. *Natural History, Clinical Spectrum, and General Management of HIV Disease* (online). Available online: http://hivinsite.ucsf.edu/akb/1997/04wom/index.html#Ab (accessed 9 August, 1999)

Newman (2004) Women and HIV. In: HIV InSite Knowledge Base Chapter (online). Available online: http://hivinsite.ucsf.edu/InSite?page=kb-03-01-12#S3.7X (accessed 9 November, 2004)

Norman AD, Perry MJ, Stevenson LY, Kelly JA and Roffman RA (1996) Lesbian and bisexual women in small cities — at risk for HIV? HIV Prevention Community Collaborative. *Public Health Rep* **111**(4): 347–52

Ocamb K, Hall J, Long I (1997) Gender matters. *POZ* **12**: 75-91

Panel on Clinical Practices for Treatment of HIV Infection convened by the DHHS (2004) *Guidelines for the Use of Antiretroviral Agents in HIV-1-Infected Adults and Adolescents* (online). Available online: http://aidsinfo.nih.gov/guidelines/default_db2.asp?id=50 (accessed 9 November, 2004)

Pillay K, Coutsoudis A, York D *et al* (2000) Cell-free virus in breast milk of HIV-1-seropositive women. *J Acquir Immune Defic Syndr* **24**: 330–6

Semprini AE, Fiore S (2004) HIV and reproduction. *Curr Opin Obstet Gynecol* **16**(3) : 257–62

Stratton P, Gupta P, Kalish L *et al* (1996) Immune status, STDs and cervical dysplasia on Pap smear in HIV+ pregnant and non-pregnant women in the Women and Infants Transmission Study (WITS). In: Program and Abstracts of the 3rd Conference on Retroviruses and Opportunistic Infections, Washington DC, A426: 133

Surgeon General (1993) Condom use for prevention of sexual transmission of HIV infection. *JAMA* **269**: 2840

Tuomala RE, Shapiro DE, Mofenson LM, Bryson Y *et al* (2002) Antiretroviral therapy during pregancy and the risk of an adverse outcome. *N Engl J Med* **346**(24): 1863–70

UK Chief Medical Officers' Expert Advisory Group on AIDS (2004) *HIV and infant feeding: Guidance from the UK Chief Medical Officers' Expert Advisory Group on AIDS*. DOH, London

Watts DH (2002) Drug therapy: management of human immunodeficiency virus infection in pregnancy. *N Engl J Med* **346**: 1879–91

Watts DH, Covington DL, Beckerman K, Garcia P, Scheuerle A, Dominguez K *et al* (2004) Assessing the risk of birth defects associated with antiretroviral exposure during pregnancy. *Am J Obstet Gynecol* **191**(3): 985–92

Weller S, Davis K (2002) Condom effectiveness in reducing heterosexual HIV transmission. The Cochrane Database of Systematic Reviews 2002, Issue 1. Art No CD003255. DOI: 10.1002/14651858.CD003255

White JC (1997) HIV risk assessment and prevention in lesbians and women who have sex with women: practical information for clinicians. *Health Care Women Int* **18**(2): 127–38

Chapter 3

HIV screening during pregnancy: ethical issues

Department of Health guidelines require midwives to offer and recommend routine HIV testing to pregnant women, along with other tests during the booking visit (NHS Executive, 1999). Various issues surrounding testing reflect the special nature of this test. This chapter will examine the midwife's role in relation to HIV screening by applying the ethical principles of beneficence, non-maleficence, autonomy, informed consent and confidentiality. Midwives should be guided by *Changing Childbirth* (DoH, 1993), which advocates a woman-centred approach to care. Women should be in control of what happens to them and able to choose the tests they want. To do this they need accurate information based on the best currently available evidence.

In 1992, the DoH advocated offering named voluntary HIV antibody testing to all women during pregnancy in areas of 'high HIV prevalence', such as London (DoH, 1992). The policy was restated in 1994 to include women who lived in lower prevalence areas (outside London) who were considered to be at 'high risk' of being infected with HIV (DoH, 1994). Despite such policies, many infections remained undetected because of poor uptake of testing. For example, in 1995 and 1996, only 23% of infections were diagnosed at the time of birth in both London and elsewhere in the UK (Intercollegiate Working Party for Enhancing Voluntary Confidential HIV Testing in Pregnancy, 1998).

By 1998 the Intercollegiate Working Party for Enhancing Voluntary Confidential HIV Testing in Pregnancy (1998) had recommended that all pregnant women receive appropriate information on HIV infection, including the risk of vertical transmission, and that HIV testing be made universally available in all antenatal clinics. Women who were considered to be at 'high risk' were strongly recommended to have the test. Examples of 'high risk' categories of women included injecting drug users, or those who came from, or travelled to, countries with high HIV prevalence. In Greater London, where the HIV seroprevalence among pregnant women was higher than elsewhere in the UK (Health Protection Agency, 2003) (*Figure 3.1*), the test was to be offered and recommended to all women who booked, as an integral part of antenatal care.

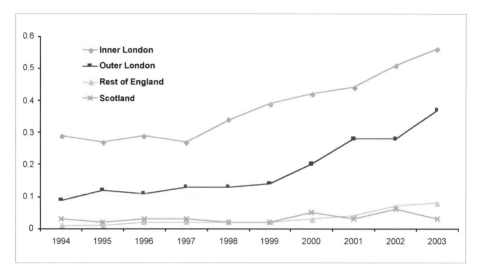

Figure 3.1: Overall prevalence[1] of HIV infection in pregnant women[2] by area of residence in England and Scotland, 1994–2003 (Health Protection Agency, 2003).

1   Tested through newborn infant dried blood spots taken for metabolic screening.
2   Includes previously diagnosed, those diagnosed through antenatal screening and those remaining undiagnosed.

Data source: unlinked anonymous serosurveillance.

Selective or universal testing?

It could be argued that the cost of offering routine screening outweighs the benefits in areas of supposedly low HIV prevalence. However, this argument has been disputed, for example, by Anthony *et al* (1992):

> *The logical inconsistency of this argument lies in the realisation that when it comes to the HIV virus, you either prevent inoculation or face the consequences of infection. Waiting until the prevalence has risen before introducing a screening programme does not solve the problem.*

Offering selective testing is a cheaper option, compared with offering universal testing. However, selective testing is the less favourable option for several reasons. For example, selective testing leads women to underestimate their risk of infection if they are not in a recognised risk group, lulling those who are perceived to be 'low risk' into a false sense of security (Catalan *et al*, 1991). Selective testing is also less effective in determining infection rates. Lindgren *et al* (1993) found that selective screening identified only 63% of seropositive patients; another study revealed that selective testing failed to detect 86% of

HIV-infected mothers (Krasinski *et al*, 1998); and two other reports found that only 58% (Landesman *et al*, 1987) and 45% (Wemstrom and Zuidema, 1989) of those identified as being seropositive had self-identified risk factors. A considerable proportion of HIV-positive women attending antenatal clinics are not aware of, or are unwilling to disclose, risky behaviour. Barbacci *et al* (1991) suggest that universal testing avoids possible stigmatisation of those identified as 'at risk'. They carried out a large study in an inner-city area of Baltimore, USA, and found that selective screening of women with identified 'risk factors' would only have detected 57% of HIV-seropositive women. When universal testing was offered to all pregnant women the detection rate was much higher (87%).

Universal testing is also the more favoured option among women. For example, one study found that only 10% of women and 6% of midwives were in favour of selective testing (Catalan *et al*, 1991). In another study, in which 789 women were asked to complete a questionnaire, of the 94% who responded, the majority (67%) agreed that HIV testing should be offered to all women (Duffy *et al*, 1998).

Women were more likely to consent to HIV testing if they were non-Caucasian, if they had thought about the test before pregnancy and if they had been seen by one particular midwife. Also, rates of testing were higher in hospital than in community clinics. Other research supports the finding that uptake of testing varies (3%–82%) depending on which midwife is offering the test (Meadows *et al*, 1990). This highlights the need for effective education for all midwives, to enable them to provide information in an unbiased way.

In the past, various factors have contributed to poor detection rates of HIV infection in pregnant women. Unfortunately, this meant that the majority of vertically infected children were only recognised as being infected when the child became symptomatic or at the time of an AIDS-defining illness (*Figure 3.2*) (PHLS, CDSC, SCIEH and ICH [L], 1999).

By 13 August 1999, the DoH had issued a press release which set out targets to cut numbers of babies born with HIV by 80% (DoH, 1999). This received coverage on national television, when Tessa Jowell, the incumbent Minister for Public Health, announced the recommendations of the Expert Group which was set up in April 1999 and chaired by the Deputy Chief Medical Officer, Dr Jeremy Metters. All women were to be offered and recommended to have an HIV test along with other tests during pregnancy. Health authorities were to be given details of targets to improve the uptake of testing to at least 50% by the end of 2000 and 90% by 2002.

The Health Service Circular (NHS Executive, 1999) raised issues for midwives who have a key role in ensuring that women are able to make an informed choice in relation to HIV testing. Midwives should be guided by the principles of *Changing Childbirth* (DoH, 1993), which advocates a 'woman-centred' approach to care. Midwives need to ensure that all women, including those from different cultural groups, are able to understand the relevant information, and that women are not coerced into having the test against their will. Midwives should be prepared to discuss the test, which involves providing accurate information based on the best currently available evidence.

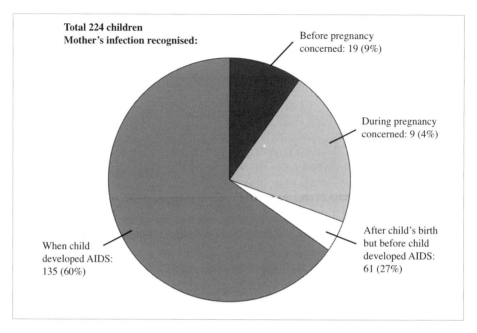

Figure 3.2: AIDS diagnoses in vertically infected children born in the UK: data to January 1999. Source: Voluntary confidential reporting by Obstetricians (RCOG), Paediatricians (BPSU/RCPCH) and Laboratories (CDSC/PHLS).

Diagnosis rates of HIV in pregnant women have increased as a result of this policy. In 2002 there were an estimated 686 births to HIV-infected women in England, Wales and Scotland, of which at least 79% (539/686) were reported as diagnosed before delivery. Estimated HIV detection rates in pregnant women have been broken down as follows:

- London — 75% (318/422)
- elsewhere in England and Wales — 85% (199/234)
- Scotland — 73% (22/30).

These minimum estimates are likely to rise as more diagnosed infections are reported (Health Protection Agency, 2003).

Better diagnosis rates for HIV infection during pregnancy are enabling infected women to make informed choices regarding interventions to reduce the risk of mother-to-child transmission (MTCT) of HIV infection from 25%–30% to less than 2% (Low-Beer and Smith, 2004). When a positive HIV antibody test result is identified, the woman is given the result by an appropriately trained healthcare professional, such as a specialist nurse or midwife, an HIV physician or an obstetrician, and information is given regarding interventions such as antiretroviral therapy, caesarean section and the avoidance of breast-feeding (Low-Beer and Smith, 2004).

The pregnant woman who is infected with HIV will need to be cared for by a multidisciplinary team consisting of an HIV physician, an obstetrician, a midwife, and a paediatrician. In addition, some women may need to be referred to a social worker, and may require the expertise of the psychiatric services. Further support and help are available to women and their families who are able to access this from voluntary organisations and support groups.

Figure 3.3 shows the potential benefits of the HIV screening programme for pregnant women in the UK. As the proportion of HIV-infected women diagnosed before delivery has increased, the proportion of infants infected with HIV has fallen. In London, in 2002, the estimated proportion of children exposed to vertical HIV transmission who became infected was 8% compared with 19% in 1997. In the rest of the UK, this proportion decreased from 22% in 1997 to 6% in 2002 (Health Protection Agency, 2003).

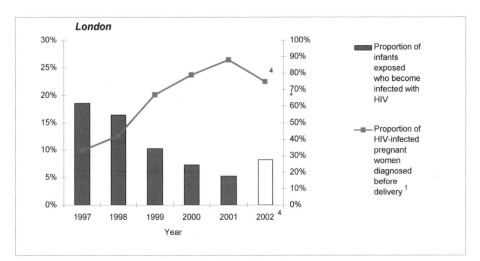

Figure 3.3: Estimated proportion of HIV-infected women diagnosed before delivery[1] and of exposed children becoming infected with HIV[2,3], 1997–2002

1   Includes those previously diagnosed and those diagnosed through antenatal testing.
2   Assumes a vertical transmission rate of 26.5% in undiagnosed women and 2.2% in diagnosed women (Duong T, Ades A, Gibb DM *et al* [1999] Vertical transmission rates for HIV in the British Isles: estimates based on surveillance data. *Br Med J* **319**: 1227–9).
3   These data contain reports received by the end of September 2003.
4   Data for 2002 should be considered preliminary minimum estimates, and as the number of reports rise, estimates of infants becoming HIV-infected will fall.
Data source: unlinked anonymous programme and the National Study of HIV in Pregnancy and Childhood (NSHPC)

HIV prevalence of women giving birth

As can be seen from *Figure 3.1*, the overall HIV prevalence of women giving birth in England and Scotland increased in 2002. London, which had a prevalence of 0.38% (422/105 817), remained the region with the greatest number of births to HIV-infected women. Between 2001 and 2002, there was a marked increase in HIV prevalence in inner London to 0.53% (251/47,075), while in outer London the prevalence remained steady at 0.29% (171/58,742). Elsewhere, the prevalence rose to 0.06% for both the rest of England (186/294,236) and Scotland (30/51,288). Overall, HIV prevalence includes those already diagnosed before pregnancy; those diagnosed through antenatal screening; and those remaining undiagnosed at delivery.

Of all women giving birth in London, an estimated 0.1% (105/105,500) had an undiagnosed HIV infection at delivery. This accounts for 25% (105/422) of all HIV infections among pregnant women in this region. Elsewhere in England and Scotland, the proportion of pregnant women with undiagnosed HIV infection was estimated to be 0.01% (33/345,341) (Health Protection Agency, 2003).

Women giving birth who were born in sub-Saharan Africa had the highest HIV prevalence with 2.47% (239/10,526) infected in 2002. The prevalence in this group of women has increased from 1.5% in 1997. Of the women born in sub-Saharan Africa, the highest prevalence occurred in those who were born in Central Africa and Eastern Africa (3.4%). Outside sub-Saharan Africa the highest prevalence of 0.37% (7/1887) was in women born in Central America and the Caribbean. Women born in the UK had a much lower prevalence of 0.03% (42/121,833), which has remained unchanged since 1997 (Health Protection Agency, 2003).

Having reflected on some of the background to HIV screening during pregnancy, ethical principals that underpin the midwife's role in relation to offering and recommending HIV testing during pregnancy will be applied (*Box 3.1*).

Box 3.1 Ethical principals
❖ Beneficence
❖ Non-maleficence
❖ Informed consent
❖ Autonomy
❖ Confidentiality

Beneficence

When applying the ethical principle of beneficence, the midwife should ensure that the outcomes of care result in 'good' being done to the woman and her baby. This entails informing women of the advantages of HIV testing during pregnancy. The benefits of HIV testing are:

Reduced rate of vertical transmission

Less than 2% of MTCTs occur during the first and second trimesters of pregnancy, whereas over 80% occur from the thirty-sixth week of pregnancy onwards, during labour and at delivery (Kourtis *et al*, 2001). The vast majority (70%) occur during labour and delivery (DeCock *et al*, 2000). The main obstetric risk factors for MTCT are vaginal delivery, prolonged duration of membrane rupture, chorioamnionitis, and pre-term delivery (European Collaborative Study, 1999).

The following interventions have been found to reduce the risk of vertical transmission.

Antiretroviral therapy

Zidovudine (also known as AZT) was the first drug approved for the treatment of HIV. The drug is in a class of drugs called nucleoside reverse transcriptase inhibitors (NRTIs). The body breaks down these drugs into chemicals that stop HIV from infecting uninfected cells in the body, but they do not help cells that have already been infected.

A randomised, double-blind, placebo-controlled trial which assessed efficacy and safety of zidovudine in reducing the risk of MTCT of HIV was done from April 1991 to December, 1993 (Conner *et al,* 1994). Four-hundred and seventy-seven HIV-infected pregnant women (fourteen to thirty-four weeks' gestation) with CD4 T-lymphocyte counts above 200 cells per cubic millimetre, who had not received antiretroviral therapy during the current pregnancy, were enrolled. During the study period, 409 gave birth to 415 live-born infants. HIV-infection status was known in 363 of the births (180 in the zidovudine group and 183 in the placebo group). Thirteen infants in the zidovudine group and forty in the placebo group were HIV-infected. The proportions infected at eighteen months were 8.3% in the zidovudine group and 25.5% in the placebo group (*Table 3.1*). This corresponds to a 67.5% reduction in the risk of HIV transmission. The researchers concluded that for pregnant women with mildly symptomatic HIV disease and no prior treatment with antiretroviral drugs, a regimen of zidovudine administered antenatally, during labour, and postnatally to the mother and the baby for six weeks, reduced the risk of maternal-infant HIV transmission by about two-thirds. This intervention was rapidly introduced in developed countries and since then, many observational studies have reported similar benefits (Low-Beer and Smith, 2004).

Current RCOG guidelines, which outline the best practice for management of HIV in pregnancy, state that maternal as well as fetal factors need to be considered when determining treatment for individual women. The guidelines recommend that women who usually have a low plasma viral load (less than 10,000–20,000 copies/ml) and a well-preserved CD4 T-lymphocyte count (greater than $350 \times 106/L$) would usually need to start antiretroviral therapy from twenty-eight to thirty-two weeks of gestation, and this should be continued intrapartum. Treatment is usually discontinued after the delivery, when considered appropriate by the HIV physician, and zidovudine is administered orally to the neonate for four to six weeks. The risk of preterm delivery will influence when antiretroviral treatment is best started, taking into account risk factors such as multiple pregnancy or a history of previous preterm labour (Low-Beer and Smith, 2004).

Table 3.1: Zidovudine (AZT) in pregnancy
Action
❖ Zidovudine is an antirectroviral drug that inhibits HIV replication   ❖ Treatment results in a significant reduction in the risk of vertical transmission from 25.5%–8.3% (Connor *et al*, 1994)
Dosage/route
❖ Oral zidovudine 100mg five times daily started between fourteen and thirty-four weeks of pregnancy   ❖ I/V zidovudine during labour, 2mg/kg body weight over a one-hour period, followed by continuous infusion of 1mg/kg/hr until delivery   ❖ Zidovudine syrup given to baby, 2mg/kg, four times a day for six weeks, beginning eight to twelve hours after delivery

One of two therapeutic options are recommended by the British HIV Association (Lyall *et al*, 2001) (*Table 3.2*).

Women with more advanced disease are more likely to have greater plasma viraemia and greater viral replication. Zidovudine, when given alone, may not effectively suppress plasma viraemia to undetectable levels. This may result in the emergence of resistant virus, which could compromise the therapeutic options available to the mother when she needs to commence treatment for her own benefit (Low-Beer and Smith, 2004).

Potent combinations of three or more antiretroviral drugs, known as HAART, have now become the standard of care for all HIV-positive women requiring antiretroviral therapy for their own health (Low-Beer and Smith, 2004). Pregnant women are treated with HAART in the same way as non-pregnant women who require HAART, usually when the CD4 T-lymphocyte count falls to $200-350 \times 10^6$/L (Lyall *et al*, 2001). Treatment should ideally start after the first trimester, and continue after the delivery of the baby.

In addition to reducing the risk of vertical transmission, zidovudine decreases the risk of infant death within the first year of birth and the risk of maternal death, while having no effect on the incidence of premature delivery or low birth weight (Brocklehurst and Volmink, 2004).

Table 3.2: Therapeutic options recommended by the British HIV Association
Option 1: A single-agent zidovudine regimen
❖ Zidovudine is given orally twice a day during pregnancy ❖ Zidovudine is given intravenously intrapartum ❖ Zidovudine is discontinued immediately after delivery ❖ Delivery should be by elective caesarean section
Benefits
❖ Exposure of the mother and fetus to larger numbers of potentially toxic drugs is avoided
Option 2: A short-term antiretroviral therapy (START) regimen
❖ HAART is given during pregnancy ❖ HAART is discontinued shortly after delivery, provided that the maternal viral load is undetectable
Benefits
❖ Maternal plasma viraemia is more likely to be suppressed to undetectable levels ❖ Fewer MTCTs are therefore envisaged ❖ Risk of the mother developing resistant virus may be lower (Low-Beer and Smith, 2004)

Bottle-feeding

MTCT can occur throughout the period of breast-feeding, although researchers have found that the risk of MTCT is influenced by breast milk virus load, which is highest early after delivery. Women who breast-fed had a significantly higher median virus load in colostrum/early milk, compared with the mature breast milk collected fourteen days after delivery (Rousseau *et al*, 2003).

Breast-feeding increases the risk of MTCT by 14% for women infected with HIV before birth, and by 30% in mothers infected postnatally (Dunn *et al*, 1992). In the UK, all women who are HIV-positive should be advised to bottle-feed their babies (Low-Beer and Smith, 2004). However, midwives need to be aware of cultural issues when advising and supporting women (*Case study*, overleaf).

> **Case study**
>
> Abisola is a twenty-four-year-old African woman who has been living in London for two years. She is fourteen weeks pregnant and HIV testing has confirmed that she is infected with HIV. Bottle-feeding has been advised in addition to other interventions. The avoidance of breast-feeding will pose problems for Abisola as her cultural background views breast-feeding as the norm. She needs to think about how she will manage to bottle-feed within her social network. Her midwife spends time with Abisola and her partner discussing various strategies for dealing with the potential dilemmas posed when bottle-feeding.

Elective caesarean section

An individual-patient meta-analysis incorporating 8533 mother-infant pairs from fifteen prospective cohort studies found that elective caesarean section decreased the risk of MTCT of HIV by more than 50%, after adjustment for antiretroviral therapy, maternal disease stage, and birthweight. Compared with other modes of delivery and no antiretroviral therapy, elective caesarean delivery and the three-part zidovudine regimen combined reduced transmission by more than 85% (International Perinatal HIV Group, 1999).

In addition, a randomised trial of mode of delivery in Europe found a transmission rate of 1%–8% among women randomly assigned to elective caesarean section compared with 10–5% for women randomly assigned to vaginal delivery. About 65% of women were taking prophylactic antiretroviral therapy (European Mode of Delivery Collaboration, 1999). Delivery by caesarean section in women taking the long course of AZT and who do not breast-feed reduces the risk of MTCT to about 1% (UNAIDS, 1999).

There is therefore good evidence to support the RCOG recommendation that HIV-positive women with a detectable plasma viral load and/or who are not taking HAART should be offered an elective caesarean section. Practice points have been summarised in *Table 3.3*. Further research is required to evaluate whether delivery by elective caesarean section has a beneficial effect on MTCT and maternal health for women who are taking HAART or who have very low viral loads, as the beneficial effect of caesarean delivery in women with viral loads of less than fifty copies/ml is uncertain (Low-Beer and Smith, 2004).

Some women may choose not to have a planned caesarean section. Women who choose a vaginal birth would benefit from discussing a birth plan with their midwife. They should be advised regarding the RCOG recommendations for managing normal labour to ensure maximal benefit and minimal harm (*Table 3.4*).

Table 3.3: RCOG guidelines for elective caesarean section (Low-Beer and Smith, 2004)

❖ The caesarean section should be planned to take place after thirty-eight weeks of gestation

❖ A zidovudine infusion should be started four hours before the caesarean section is begun

❖ The cord should be clamped as soon as possible after the baby is delivered

---

Table 3.4: RCOG guidelines for a planned vaginal delivery (Low-Beer and Smith, 2004)

❖ Membranes should be left intact for as long as possible

❖ Use of fetal scalp electrode and fetal blood sampling should be avoided

❖ Women should continue their HAART regime throughout labour

❖ If an intravenous infusion of zidovudine is required, it should be started at the beginning of labour

❖ The infusion should be continued until the cord is clamped

❖ The cord should be clamped as soon as possible after the baby is delivered

❖ A maternal blood sample should be taken at delivery, and tested for plasma viral load

❖ The baby should be bathed immediately after the birth

Other interventions that may further reduce the risk of MTCT include:

⌘ **The avoidance of invasive prenatal procedures** (Anastos *et al*, 1997). However, evidence regarding the risks of MTCT with chorionic villus sampling or second-trimester amniocentesis is lacking, and RCOG guidelines state that when such procedures are contemplated, the advice of the HIV physician and the fetal medicine specialist should be sought. If invasive prenatal testing is undertaken, prophylaxis with HAART should be considered (Low-Beer and Smith, 2004).

⌘ **Screening and treatment of other sexually transmitted infections.** RCOG guidelines recommend that women who are HIV-positive should be offered screening for genital infections as early as possible in pregnancy, and again at twenty-eight weeks of pregnancy (Low-Beer and Smith, 2004). This includes testing for *Chlamydia trachomatis*, *Neisseria gonorrhoea*, bacterial vaginosis, syphilis, hepatitis B and hepatitis C. The rationale is that the majority of pregnant women in the UK who are HIV-positive come from sub-Saharan Africa, where the prevalence of genital infections is high. In addition, organisms associated with bacterial vaginosis have been shown to stimulate HIV *in-vitro*, and preliminary data suggest that bacterial vaginosis may be associated with an increased risk of MTCT (Taha *et al*, 1998). Screening and treatment of genital tract infections is therefore beneficial, as it may further reduce the incidence of MTCT as well as improve maternal health outcomes.

Benefits for the mother

Early diagnosis of HIV enables 'optimal control' of HIV infection, improving maternal health and life expectancy. This is achieved when a woman with a measurable viral burden consistently adheres to taking HAART, has a stable or increasing CD4 count, is receiving appropriate prophylaxis for opportunistic infections, based on the lowest past CD4 count, and has achieved maximal suppression of HIV replication load (Beckerman, 1998).

Women will benefit from having their plasma viral load and CD4 T-lymphocyte measurements reviewed at regular intervals, and from being given advice regarding the choice and timing of antiretroviral therapy and the need for prophylaxis of *Pneumocystis carinii* pneumonia. Co-trimoxazole, the drug of choice for *Pneumocystis carinii* pneumonia prophylaxis, is usually administered when the CD4 T-lymphocyte count is below 200x106/L (Low-Beer and Smith, 2004).

Blood testing to assess the full blood count, urea and electrolytes, liver function, lactate and glucose levels will enable women who are taking antiretroviral drugs to be monitored for drug toxicities. They are also offered a detailed ultrasound scan to detect fetal anomalies. In particular, the detection of fetal anomalies potentially attributable to teratogenesis after first-trimester exposure to HAART, and folate antagonists used for prophylaxis against PCP (Low-Beer and Smith, 2004) in women who are diagnosed HIV-positive prior to becoming pregnant, may be beneficial. Women who become pregnant and are already receiving combination antiretroviral therapy are advised to continue their therapy, as any interruption is likely to be associated with rebound of plasma HIV RNA measurements to pre-treatment levels or higher (Beckerman, 1998). As both HIV disease and pregnancy place major nutritional burdens on women's bodies (Beckerman, 1998), they should be referred to a dietician.

Offering the test gives a valuable opportunity to provide health education for all women to enable them to understand how the HIV virus is transmitted and how infection can be prevented. Ensuring women receive effective health education is important, as diagnoses of HIV and the major acute STIs continue to rise across the UK, and the high risk behaviours which drive the transmission are also on the increase (Health Protection Agency, 2003).

A review of the literature concerning the effectiveness of health education at informing young people about HIV and AIDS has revealed that there are gaps in young people's knowledge base, and there is still a reluctance to use condoms (Gilbert, 1994). Many of the studies reported that AIDS was still seen as a disease of high-risk category groups rather than of the heterosexual community. In two studies, most of the respondents had no understanding that AIDS could be contracted from an asymptomatic carrier (Kaul and Stephens, 1991; Petosa and Wessinger, 1990; cited by Gilbert, 1994). These findings are cause for concern and a challenge to midwives who should be able to clarify any misconceptions.

Benefits for the baby

It has been estimated from the National Study of HIV in Pregnancy and Childhood (NSHPC), that by the end of June 2003, 3576 children were born to HIV-infected women in the UK: 998 (28%) of these babies were infected and 1700 (48%) were uninfected. The infection status of the remainder was unreported or unresolved. Cumulative data to the end of December 2002 show that 188 children under the age of fourteen, who acquired HIV infection from their mother died (Health Protection Agency, 2003).

Most babies initially have antibodies to HIV as a result of the transfer of maternal antibodies across the placenta. These antibodies disappear by eighteen months in babies who have not become infected. Most cases of paediatric HIV infection are diagnosed by one month of age using sensitive viral tests, while virtually all are diagnosable by six months (Josefson 1997). Direct viral amplification by polymerase chain reaction is usually done at birth, then at three weeks, six weeks and six months. Over 99% of non-breast-fed babies who have a negative HIV test result by polymerase chain reaction at six months will be uninfected. The definitive test is the HIV antibody test, and a negative result at eighteen months of age will confirm that the child is uninfected (Low-Beer and Smith, 2004).

Treating the babies of mothers who received zidovudine antenatally and intrapartum, either as single-agent therapy or as part of a HAART regimen, reduces the risk of mother-to-child transmission. Zidovudine is started at birth and should be discontinued after four to six weeks unless the mother started antiretroviral therapy late in pregnancy (within four weeks of delivery). According to expert opinion, HAART may be considered if the mother started antiretroviral therapy late in pregnancy. However, for preterm or sick neonates who are unable to tolerate oral medication, zidovudine is the only preparation that may be given intravenously (Lyall *et al*, 2001).

In the past, about 30%–50% of HIV-infected children presented with an early onset of opportunistic infections such as *Pneumocystis carinii* pneumonia, while those that did better had no signs or symptoms of disease until eight to ten years of age (Scarlatti, 1996). Without treatment, approximately 23%–26% of HIV-infected babies will develop features characteristic of AIDS within the first year of life, and their health will deteriorate rapidly (Scarlatti, 1996).

However, all infants with confirmed HIV infection who are under twelve months of age should now be treated with combination antiretroviral therapy (Josefson, 1997). HIV-infected children benefit from treatment in the same way as HIV-infected adults, although because infants who acquire the infection perinatally are still developing their immune system during the first six months of life, they have potentially more to gain from such treatment (Josefson, 1997).

The benefits of treatment of children with perinatally acquired HIV infection in the UK have been well documented. Data from national obstetric and paediatric surveillance registers showed that by January 1999, the proportion of infected children developing AIDS within the first six months of life fell from 17.7% before 1994 to 7.2% from 1994 onwards, coinciding with increased use of prophylaxis against *Pneumocystis carinii* pneumonia (Duong *et al*, 1999).

Since the introduction of three- or four-drug antiretroviral therapy in 1997, mortality, AIDS, and hospital admission rates have declined substantially in the UK and Ireland. Mortality decreased by 80% between 1997 and 2001–2, paralleling the increased use of three- and four-drug combination antiretroviral therapy; AIDS progression decreased by 50% and hospital admission rates decreased by 80%. Most reductions occurred in 1997–9, with rates stabilising between 2000 and 2002 (Gibb *et al*, 2003).

Benefits for the family

Informed decisions can be made regarding the current pregnancy, the planning of future pregnancies, and testing other family members for HIV. The woman, possibly in consultation with her partner, will be able to make an informed choice regarding continuation of the pregnancy, although research has shown that knowledge of HIV seropositivity and the subsequent decision to terminate the pregnancy is not often made on the basis of testing positive (Johnstone and Brettle, 1990). Advice can also be given in relation to preventing the spread of HIV infection.

Non-maleficence

When applying the ethical principle of non-maleficence, the midwife should ensure that any act or omission does not result in harm. An awareness of any potential 'harm' (*Box 3.2*) will enable midwives to discuss individual concerns with women, who must decide for themselves whether screening is in their best interests. Midwives can also offer advice and support to minimise any potential harm associated with the management of HIV infection. To provide optimal care, midwives need to be knowledgeable about the potential effects of different treatments.

> **Box 3.2: Potential 'harm'**
>
> ❖ Adverse consequences of a negative result
> ❖ Psychological impact — suicide risk
> ❖ Social sequelae — impact on work/family/relationships
> ❖ Stigma/discrimination
> ❖ Insurance/mortgage issues (if positive)
> ❖ Unnecessary treatment of about 85% of mothers and their
>   uninfected babies
> ❖ Side-effects of antiretroviral therapy
> ❖ Potentially increased risk of pre-eclampsia
> ❖ Risks associated with sepsis following caesarean section are
>   greater in HIV-infected women
> ❖ Avoidance of breast-feeding

Possible adverse consequences of a negative result

A negative result may have adverse consequences because of what has been described as the 'certificate of health effect' (Tymstra and Bieleman, 1987). The individual is inclined to regard a negative test result as justification for an unhealthy lifestyle and therefore deny the need to change.

Women should also be made aware that the HIV test detects antibodies that are present in the woman's blood at that time. A woman who thinks she may have recently been exposed to HIV infection may want to be re-tested later in pregnancy, which should be arranged for her as the first negative test result does not guarantee against newly-acquired infection (DoH, RCM, 1999).

Psychological impact — suicide risk

Awaiting the results of an HIV test and receiving a positive result can be highly stressful, and midwives need to be sensitive to a woman's need for support. Receiving an HIV diagnosis is traumatic, and reactions of shock, fear and anguish have been reported (Stevens and Tighe, 1997). According to Campbell (1995), many people commit suicide while awaiting HIV test results, or upon receiving a positive diagnosis, or at a later stage of disease progression.

Researchers investigating the experiences of women being informed of a positive HIV antibody test found that they often experienced unrelenting misery; for some, the shadow of death hung over them thereafter. The thought of potentially causing death to others was also common. For example, one woman said, 'When I found out... my baby had AIDS, I was thinking, he is going to die. What if he dies? O God, I am a murderer. What have I done?' (Stevens and Tighe, 1997).

Social sequelae — impact on work/family/relationships

After testing positive for HIV, women often experience unrelenting misery, escalating drug use and transmission risks, and destabilisation of relationships, income and shelter (Stevens and Tighe, 1997). Other examples of harm include risk of rejection, isolation and domestic violence (Lester *et al*, 1995). Midwives must therefore refer women to specialist counsellors and social workers to reduce the potential social and psychological 'harm'.

Midwives can also give details of HIV support groups to a woman when she is diagnosed (*Reader activity*). Women and their families may benefit from many of the services provided by such organisations (*Reader activity*). Positively Women is a national charity that aims to improve the quality of life of women and families affected by HIV. It was established in 1987 by a group of HIV-positive women who were determined to set up services specific to women's needs. The women formed a support group to talk openly about the challenges they faced. Today, the organisation remains strongly committed to the ethos of peer support and empowerment by:

- providing specialist support by women living with HIV
- enabling women to make informed choices
- challenging stigma and discrimination.

Further information is available from their website: www.ukcoalition.org.

Reader activity

- ❖ Identify appropriate HIV support groups (voluntary agencies) for women in your area, including contact details and referral information
- ❖ Identify the ways in which women and their families may benefit from accessing such organisations

---

Stigma/discrimination

Many people who are HIV-positive still suffer discrimination and harassment. For example, there is evidence that neonatal unit staff have deliberately undertreated babies who are (or believed to be) HIV-positive (Levin, 1991). In midwifery, there is some evidence of discriminatory practice, particularly among midwives outside London (*Chapter 5*).

Insurance/mortgage issues (if positive)

There is some concern about the response of insurance companies towards people who have been tested for HIV. The Association of British Insurers has stated that routine antenatal testing is no bar to insurance and will not affect premiums. However, women who are diagnosed as HIV-positive may face disadvantages, such as difficulty in obtaining life insurance and mortgages.

Unnecessary treatment of mothers and babies

Informing women of the 15%–20% risk of vertical transmission is the same as telling them that 80%–85% of babies will not be infected. Therefore, the majority of mothers who accept the interventions on offer will be exposing themselves and their babies to unnecessary treatment (RCOG, 1997).

Side-effects of antiretroviral therapy and *Pneumocystis carinii* pneumonia prophylaxis

Zidovudine is associated with a higher incidence of neonatal anaemia (haemoglobin concentration of less than 9g/dl), although by twelve weeks of age this effect is no longer apparent (Connor *et al*, 1994). More serious side-effects have not been reported. For example, an interim report of the International Antiretroviral Pregnancy Registry, to which all women taking antiretroviral therapy in pregnancy are reported, did not find any increase in the rate of fetal anomalies (Wilmington, 2002). However, continued prospective evaluations of children born to HIV-infected women are critical to assess the long-term safety, as data from animal studies show the potential for transplacental carcinogenicity of zidovudine (Olivero *et al*, 1997).

The hypothetical findings of one study support the link between mitochondrial dysfunction and the perinatal administration of zidovudine and lamivudine. The researchers concluded that zidovudine monotherapy should continue to be recommended, and that further assessment of the toxic effects of combination therapy is needed (Blanch *et al*, 1999).

Co-trimoxazole, the drug of choice for *Pneumocystis carinii* pneumonia prophylaxis, is a folate antagonist, and administration during the first trimester may cause an increased risk of neural-tube defects. A multicentre retrospective study of 195 mother–infant pairs showed that, compared with infants not exposed to antiretroviral therapy or folate antagonists during the first trimester (n=148), exposure to both antiretroviral therapy and folate antagonists during the first trimester (n=13) produced an increased risk of congenital abnormalities (4% versus 23.1%), including one case of spina bifida. There was no evidence of teratogenicity associated with antiretroviral therapy if given alone

(Jungmann *et al*, 2001). The limitations of this study are the small sample size, and the absence of information on folic-acid supplementation and exposure to other medications, including illegal drugs. This study is not relevant to women diagnosed during pregnancy, as most women diagnosed after routine screening will be asymptomatic and will have progressed past the first trimester without any exposure to *Pneumocystis carinii* pneumonia prophylaxis. For women infected with HIV before pregnancy, and who require *Pneumocystis carinii* pneumonia prophylaxis during the first trimester of pregnancy, the health needs of the mother must be balanced against the potential harm to the fetus.

Midwives are required to provide care and advice to women, including preventative measures, and have an important task in health education and health counselling (NMC, 2002). Midwives should therefore help ensure that all women are aware of the recommended advice about folic-acid supplementation to reduce their risk of having a baby with a neural-tube defect. For example, in 1992, an Expert Committee of the Department of Health recommended that all women should increase their intake of folic acid before conceiving a child and during the first twelve weeks of pregnancy. Women can do this by:

- eating foods fortified with folic acid such as some breakfast cereals and breads
- eating foods naturally rich in folic acid, such as leafy green vegetables
- taking a daily 400mg folic acid supplement from the time they stop using contraception until the twelfth week of pregnancy.

(DoH, 1998)

Potentially increased risk of pre-eclampsia

Some evidence suggests that pre-eclampsia is more common in women taking HAART compared with those not taking antiretroviral therapy (Wimalasundera *et al*, 2002). Lactic acid acidosis, a recognised complication of HAART may mimic the signs of pre-eclampsia. Midwives therefore need to be vigilant when looking for signs of pre-eclampsia, and refer to the obstetrician for liver function tests and blood lactate monitoring where necessary. Signs of lactic acidosis include gastrointestinal disturbances, fatigue, fever and breathlessness. Other antiretroviral toxicities include hepatoxicity, rashes, glucose intolerance and diabetes, and mild self-limiting anaemia is a common side-effect of zidovudine (Low-Beer and Smith, 2004).

Risks associated with sepsis following caesarean section

The risks associated with sepsis following caesarean section are greater in HIV-infected women (UNAIDS, 1999). According to the findings of a randomised controlled trial comparing the clinical outcomes of sixty-two HIV-infected women who underwent caesarean section between 1987 and 1999, postoperative complications were significantly more common in HIV-positive women compared with HIV-negative matches. HIV-infected women were more likely to require blood transfusions, as they frequently developed anaemia, and postpartum pyrexia requiring antibiotics was especially common (Grubert *et al*, 1999). However, in the randomised trial of mode of delivery in Europe, there were few postpartum complications and no serious adverse events in either group (European Mode of Delivery Collaboration, 1999).

Avoidance of breast-feeding

The WHO recommendation that HIV-infected women who have access to safe artificial feeding methods should avoid breast-feeding, while those living in areas where artificial feeding may be unsafe because of unclean water supplies should breast-feed their infants, is based on relatively few studies of poor quality (Brocklehurst, 2004). One study of 549 HIV-infected women found that exclusive breast-feeding carries a significantly lower risk of HIV transmission (almost half the risk) than mixed feeding and a similar risk to no breast-feeding (Coutsoudis *et al*, 1999). The researchers suggest that HIV acquired during delivery may become neutralised by immune factors present in breast milk but not in formula feeds. They also point out that breast milk contains growth factors, such as epidermal growth factor and transforming growth factor ß, which may enhance maturation of the gut epithelial barrier, thus maintaining its integrity and hindering passage of the virus (Udall, 1981; Planchon *et al*, 1994). It is believed that in the mixed feeding group, the beneficial immune factors of breast milk are probably counteracted by damage to the infant's gut by contaminants or allergens in mixed feeds. Further research is required to confirm or elucidate these findings.

In the UK, some women may choose to breast-feed despite the risk of mother-to-child transmission This scenario obviously poses complex child protection issues for healthcare professionals. According to Leroy *et al* (1998), if HIV-infected women choose to breast-feed, they should be advised to avoid giving any other foods for at least the first three months. Early and abrupt weaning should be advised because of the increased risk of late postnatal transmission through breast milk after three to six months, and because introduction of other foods becomes more frequent as the infant gets older.

The administration of antiretroviral drugs to breast-feeding women throughout the period of breast-feeding would provide optimal prevention of mother-to-child transmission. However, it has been argued that the long-term efficacy of antiretroviral prophylaxis is limited because of the potential toxic effects, the development of drug resistance and the relatively short half-life (Safrit *et al*, 2004). In the future, a safe and effective active/passive immunoprophylaxis regimen, begun at birth, and potentially overlapping with intrapartum or neonatal chemoprophylaxis, could potentially be a more effective strategy (Safrit *et al*, 2004).

HIV is a complex pathogen, and although maternal antibodies capable of traversing the placenta and present in breast milk play an important part in protecting neonates from many bacterial and viral pathogens, finding a vaccine that contains antibodies capable of neutralising a wide array of primary HIV isolates has been problematic, according to Safrit *et al* (2004). However, several unique monoclonal antibodies that can neutralise many isolates of HIV have been derived from HIV-infected humans. It is mainly these potent examples of anti-HIV monoclonal antibodies that have given potential passive immunoprophylaxis protocols new life, and several successful experiments in animal models provide strong supporting data that passive administration of antibodies can prevent HIV infection. In the near future, trials should begin to determine whether pregnant women can be given vaccines that generate such antibody responses, and whether vaccine-induced maternal neutralising antibodies can cross the placenta (Safrit *et al*, 2004).

The WHO/UNAIDS HIV Vaccine Initiative was established in 2000 to facilitate the development and evaluation of appropriate HIV vaccines, ensuring that once they are developed they are affordable and available to all people in need. According to the WHO and UNAIDS, recent HIV vaccine trial results are an important step forward in developing an effective vaccine (WHO, 2004).

Informed consent

Each woman needs to be aware of the implications of receiving an HIV diagnosis so that she can decide for herself whether testing would be in her best interest and, if necessary, make informed decisions about treatment and interventions. According to Gillon (1986), 'consent is given when an individual makes a voluntary uncoerced decision on the basis of adequate information and deliberation'. Midwives should ensure that women are provided with relevant and up-to-date information in an appropriate way (*Box 3.3*). The 'information should be accurate, truthful and presented in such a way as to make it easily understood' (NMC, 2002).

Leaflets can be useful and, if sent to the woman before the booking interview, may serve as a basis for discussion before testing. Some women may require more time to consider the implications before making their decision, and midwives should offer a further appointment in such instances.

To provide a 'woman-centred' approach to care, midwives must ensure that all women, including those from different cultural groups, are able to understand the relevant information (*Reader activity*).

In a study by Duffy *et al* (1998), midwives gave women a leaflet and information about HIV infection. Of the 789 (94%) who responded by completing a questionnaire, non-Caucasian women and women with lower educational qualifications had lower knowledge scores. Relevant information, therefore, must be targeted appropriately using videos and specially designed leaflets to meet the needs of different groups of women. Some hospitals have produced leaflets in different languages, including Somali, French, Bengali, Gujarati, Vietnamese and Turkish, to meet the needs of the women in their catchment area. However, knowledge does not appear to increase the uptake of testing, as 64% of women did not change their original pre-discussion decision regarding the test (Duffy *et al*, 1998).

Reader activity

❖ What care provision exists for women from ethnic minority groups?
❖ What cultural factors need to be considered when helping women (and their partners) to make an informed choice in relation to testing and management options?

Box 3.3: Information for women

❖ Nature and purpose of test
❖ Advantages
❖ Disadvantages
❖ Insurance/mortgage issues
❖ Assurance that it is a non-discriminatory service
❖ Confidentiality policy
❖ Advice on safer sex
❖ Unlinked anonymous surveys
❖ Process of testing/informing of results
❖ Risk assessment

(Antenatal HIV Testing Working Party, 1998)

Autonomy

Autonomy is inextricably linked with consent and entails facilitating a woman's ability to formulate and carry out her own plans so that she is in control of her life and can act freely within the context of rational decision-making (Downie and Calman, 1987). Midwives should ensure that women do not feel coerced into having the test, as this would cause 'harm' if the woman's rights were infringed and would also undermine the woman's sense of being in control. It may also discourage some women from seeking antenatal care. The Nursing and Midwifery Council's *Code of Professional Conduct* states that midwives must 'respect patients' and clients' autonomy — their right to decide whether or not to undergo any health care intervention — even where a refusal may result in harm or death to themselves or a fetus, unless a court of law orders to the contrary' (NMC, 2002: 4).

However, there may be attitudinal barriers to testing and treatment of HIV, which may be overcome as midwives allow time for discussion as necessary. For example, one study found that negative attitudes towards AZT were widely prevalent. Women perceived the drug as highly toxic, as prescribed indiscriminately, as inadequately tested in women and minorities, as promoted for the wrong reasons and as inappropriate while they were feeling well (Siegel and Gorey, 1997). Midwives should explore the woman's feelings, identify individual needs, and plan care in partnership with the woman. Whatever the final decision, the midwife should record in the woman's notes that the test has been offered (DoH, RCM, 1999). When obtaining consent, midwives must ensure that all discussions are documented in the woman's case notes and those who consent may do so in writing, verbally or by co-operation (NMC, 2002).

Confidentiality

A breach of confidentiality is particularly serious for women who are HIV-positive because of the risk of discrimination even within the Health Service. Midwives must 'treat information about patients and clients as confidential and use it only for the purposes for which it was given', and, 'ensure that patients and clients understand that some information may be made available to other members of the team involved in the delivery of care' (NMC, 2002: 7). In addition, midwives must 'guard against breaches of confidentiality by protecting information from improper disclosure at all times' (NMC, 2002: 7) (*Reader activity*).

Reader activity

❖ Refer to your local trust policy for midwives offering and recommending HIV screening during pregnancy.
❖ What guidelines have been included to ensure that confidentiality is maintained?
❖ Are these effective?
❖ If not, what improvements could be made?
❖ Are these effective?
❖ If not, what improvements could be made?
❖ What support and care is offered to women who have a positive test result?

In rare instances, midwives may be required to disclose information, that will have personal consequences for the woman concerned, to people outside the team. The team includes the woman, the woman's family, informal carers and health and social care professionals in the National Health Service, the independent and voluntary sectors. In such cases, midwives must obtain the consent of the woman concerned. If consent cannot be obtained, disclosures can only be made if:

- they are required by law or by order of a court
- they can be justified in the public interest (for example, to protect the woman or anyone else from significant harm) (NMC, 2002).

Where there is an issue of child protection, midwives 'must act at all times in accordance with local and national policies' (NMC, 2002; 8).

Conclusion

HIV screening during pregnancy enables infected women to benefit from interventions that are known to improve health outcomes for women and their families. Women must be given relevant information that is accurate. It must be presented in a way that makes it easy for individual women to understand. Midwives must respect women's right to decide whether or not to undergo any healthcare intervention. The rights of women must also be protected in relation to confidentiality, although some information may be made available to other members of the team involved in the delivery of care. Excellence in care provision should be the experience of all women, who are entitled to a full range of confidential services, enabling them to achieve maximum benefit and suffer minimum harm.

References

Anastos K, Denenberg R, Solomon L (1997) Human immunodeficiency virus infection in women. *Med Clin N Am* **81**(2): 533–53

Antenatal HIV Testing Working Party (1998) *Quality framework for HIV testing services in London.* Inner London HIV Health Commissioners Group, London

Anthony J, Malan A, Buccimazza S *et al* (1992) Antenatal screening for HIV infection. *South African Med J* **82**: 75–6

Barbacci M *et al* (1991) Routine prenatal screening for HIV infection. *Lancet* **337**: 709–11

Beckerman KP (1998) Reproduction and HIV disease: Pregnancy and perinatal care of HIV infected women. In: Cohen PT, ed. *Natural History, Clinical Spectrum, and General Management of HIV Disease* (online). Available online: http://hivinsite.ucsf.edu/akb/1997/04preg/index.html (accessed 4 September, 1999)

Blanche S, Tardieu M, Rustin P, Slama A, Barret B, Firtion G *et al* (1999) Persistent mitochondrial dysfunction and perinatal exposure to antiretroviral nucleoside analogues. *Lancet* **354**(9184): 1084–9

Brocklehurst P (2004) Interventions for reducing the risk of mother-to-child transmission of HIV infection (Cochrane Review). In: The Cochrane Library, Issue 3. John Wiley and Sons Ltd, Chichester

Brocklehurst P and Volmink J (2004) Antiretrovirals for reducing the risk of mother-to-child transmission of HIV infection (Cochrane Review). In: The Cochrane Library, Issue 3, 2004. John Wiley and Sons Ltd, Chichester

Campbell J (1995) HIV and suicide: is there a relationship? *AIDS Care* **7**(suppl 2): s107–s108

Catalan J, Meadows J, Stone Y, Barton S *et al* (1991) Antenatal testing for HIV. *Br Med J* **302**: 1400

Connor EM, Sperling RS, Gelber R *et al* for The Pediatric AIDS Clinical Trials Group Protocol 076 Study Group (1994) Reduction of maternal-infant transmission of human immunodeficiency virus type 1 with Zidovudine treatment. *N Engl J Med* **331**(18): 1173–80

Coutsoudis A, Pillay K, Spooner E Kuhn L, Coovadia HM for the South African Vitamin A Study Group (1999) Influence of infant-feeding patterns on early mother-to-child transmission of HIV in Durban, South Africa: a prospective cohort study. *Lancet* **354**(9177): 471

DeCock KM, Fowler MG, Mercier G *et al* (2000) Prevention of mother-to-child transmission in resource-poor countries. *JAMA 283*:1175–82

Department of Health (1992) *Offering voluntary named HIV antibody testing to women receiving antenatal care*. DoH, London

Department of Health (1994) *Guidelines for offering voluntary named HIV anti-body testing to women receiving ante-natal care*. DoH, London

Department of Health (1993) *Changing Childbirth*. HMSO, London

Department of Health (1998) Folic Acid Campaign Wins Award (online). Available online: http://www.dh.gov.uk/PublicationsAndStatistics/PressReleases (accessed 10 July, 2004)

Department of Health (1999) *Targets to cut numbers of babies born with HIV by 80% by 2002* (online). Available online: http://www.nds.coi.gov.uk/coi/coipress.nsf (accessed 2 September, 1999)

Department of Health, Royal College of Midwives (RCM) (1999) *Information for midwives. HIV testing in pregnancy*. RCM, London

Downie RS, Calman KC (1987) *Health Respect — Ethics in Health Care*. Faber and Faber, London

Duffy TA, Wolfe CDA, Varden C, Kennedy J, Chrystie IL (1998) Women's knowledge and attitudes, and the acceptability of voluntary antenatal HIV testing. *Br J Obstet Gynaecol* **105**: 849–54

Dunn DT, Newell ML, Ades AE, Peckham CS (1992) Risk of human immunodeficiency virus type 1 transmission through breast-feeding. *Lancet* **340**(8819): 585–8

Duong T, Ades AE, Gibb DM, Tookey PA, Masters J (1999) Vertical transmission rates for HIV in the British Isles: estimates based on surveillance data. *Br Med J* **319**(7219): 1227–9

European Collaborative Study (1999) Risk factors for mother-to-child transmission of HIV. *Lancet* **339**: 1007–12

European Mode of Delivery Collaboration (1999) Elective caesarean section versus vaginal delivery in prevention of vertical HIV transmission: a randomised clinical trial. *Lancet* **353**(9158): 1035–9

Gibb DM, Duong T, Tookey PA, Sharland M, Tudor-Williams G, Novelli V *et al* (2003) Decline in mortality, AIDS, and hospital admissions in perinatally HIV infected children in the United Kingdom and Ireland. *Br Med J* **327**: 1019–25

Gilbert S (1994) Is the message getting across? Effectiveness of health education at informing young people about HIV and AIDS. *Prof Nurse* **9**(11): 765–9

Gillon R (1986) *Philosophical Medical Ethics*. Wiley and Sons, Chichester

Grubert TA, Reindell D, Kästner R, Lutz-Friedrich R, Belohradsky BH *et al* (1999) Complications after caesarean section in HIV-infected women not taking antiretroviral treatment. *Lancet* **354**(9190): 1612

Health Protection Agency, SCIEH, ISD, National Public Health Service for Wales, CDSC Northern Ireland and the UASSG (2003) *Renewing the focus. HIV and other Sexually Transmitted Infections in the United Kingdom in 2002*. Health Protection Agency, London

International Perinatal HIV Group (1999) Mode of delivery and the risk of vertical transmission of human immunodeficiency virus type 1— a meta-analysis of 15 prospective cohort studies. *N Eng J Med* **340**(13): 977–87

Intercollegiate Working Party for Enhancing Voluntary Confidential HIV Testing in Pregnancy (1998) *Reducing mother-to-child transmission of HIV infection in the United Kingdom*. Executive summary and recommendations. Royal College of Paediatrics and Child Health, London

Johnstone F, Brettle R (1990) Women's knowledge of their HIV antibody. *Br Med J* **300**: 23–4

Josefson D (1997) HIV treatment in children brought into line with that in adults. *Br Med J* **315**(7113): 902

Jungmann EM, Mercey D, DeRuiter A, Edwards S, Donoghue S, Booth T *et al* (2001) Is first trimester exposure to the combination of antiretroviral therapy and folate antagonists a risk factor for congenital abnormalities? *Sex Transm Infect* **77**: 441–3

Kaul R, Stephens J (1991) AIDS, knowledge, attitudes and reported sexual behaviour among students in West Glamorgan. *Health Educ J* **50**(3): 128–30

Krasinski K, Borkowsy W, Bebenroth D, Moore T (1988) Failure of voluntary testing for HIV to identify infected parturiant women in a high risk population. *New Engl J Med* **318**: 185

Kourtis AP, Bulterys M, Nesheim SR, Lee FK (2001) Understanding the timing of HIV transmission from mother to infant. *JAMA* **285**: 709–12

Landesman S, Minkoff H, Holman S, McCalla S, Sijin O (1987) Serosurvey of HIV infection in parturiants. *JAMA* **258**: 2701–3

Leroy V, Newell ML, Dabis F *et al* (1998) International multicentre pooled analysis of late postnatal mother-to-child transmission of HIV infection. *Lancet* **352**(9128): 597–600

Lester P, Partridge JC, Chesney MA *et al* (1995) The consequences of a positive prenatal HIV antibody test for women. *J Acquired Immunodeficiency Syndrome* **10**(3): 341–9

Levin B, Driscoll J, FleischmanA, MacCullum L (1991) Treatment choices for infants in the neonatal intensive care units at risk of AIDS. *JAMA* **265**: 2976

Lindgren S *et al* (1993) Screening for HIV antibodies in pregnancy: results from the Swedish national programme. *Br Med J* **307**: 1447–51

Low-Beer NM, Smith JR (2004) *Management of HIV in Pregnancy*. RCOG Guideline No 39. Royal College of Obstetricians and Gynaecologists (online). Available online: http://www.rcog.org.uk/guidelines (accessed 30 June, 2004)

Lyall EG, Blott M, de Ruiter A, Hawkins D, Mercy D, Mitchla Z *et al* (2001) Guidelines for the management of HIV infection in pregnant women and the prevention of mother-to-child transmission. *HIV Med* **2**: 314–34

Meadows J, Jenkinson S, Catalan J, Chrystie IL, Tilzey AJ, Wolfe C (1990) Voluntary HIV testing in the antenatal clinic: differing uptake rates for individual counselling midwives. *Aids Care* **2**: 229–33

NHS Executive (1999) *Reducing mother-to-baby transmission of HIV*. Health Service Circular 1999/183. DoH, London

Nursing and Midwifery Council (NMC) (2002) *Code of Professional Conduct*. NMC, London

Olivero OA, Anderson LM, Diwan BA *et al* (1997) Transplacental effects of 3'-azido-2',3'-dideoxythymidine (AZT): tumorigenicity in mice and genotoxicity in mice and monkeys. *J Natl Cancer Inst* **89**(21): 1602–88

Petosa R, Wessinger J (1990) The AIDS educational needs of adolescents: a theory based approach. *AIDS Education and Prevention* **2**(2):127–36

Public Health Laboratory Service (PHLS) Communicable Disease Surveillance Centre (CDSC), Scottish Centre for Infection and Environmental Health (SCIEH) and Institute of Child Health (London) (ICH (L) (1999) PHLS CDSC HIV/AIDS CORE SLIDE SET (online). Available online: http://www.phls.co.uk/facts/hivslide.htm (accessed 15 December, 1999)

Planchon SM, Martins CAP, Guerrant RL, Roche JK (1994) Regulation of intestinal epithelial barrier function. *J Immunol* **153**(12): 5730–9

Royal College of Obstetrics and Gynaecology (1997) *HIV Infection in Maternity Care*. Working Party Report. RCOG Press, London

Rousseau CM, Nduati RW, Richardson BA, Steele MS, John-Stewart GC, Mbori-Ngacha DA *et al* (2003) Longitudinal analysis of human immunodeficiency virus type 1 RNA in breast milk and of its relationship to infant infection and maternal disease. *J Infect Dis 187*(5):741–7

Safrit JT, Ruprecht R, Ferrantelli F, Xu W, Kitabwalla M, Rompay KV *et al* for the Ghent IAS Working Group on HIV in Women and Children (2004) Immunoprophylaxis to prevent mother-to-child transmission of HIV. *J Acquired Immune Deficiency Syndrome* **35**(2):169–77)

Scarlatti G (1996) Paediatric HIV infection. *Lancet* **348**(9031): 863–8

Siegel K, Gorey E (1997) HIV-infected women: barriers to AZT use. *Soc Sci Med* **45**(1): 15–22

Stevens PE, Tighe Doerr B (1997) Trauma of discovery: women's narratives of being informed they are HIV infected. *Aids Care* **9**(5): 523–38

Taha TE, Hoover DR, Dallabetta GA, Kumwenda NI, Mtimavalye LA, Yang LP *et al* (1998) Bacterial vaginosis and disturbances of vaginal flora: association with increased acquisition of HIV. *AIDS* **12**: 1699–706

Tymstra T, Bieleman B (1987) The psychological impact of mass screening for cardiovascular risk factors. *Fam Practice* **4**: 287–90

Udall JN, Colony P, Fritze L, Pang K, Trier JS, Walker WA (1981) Development of gastrointestinal mucosal barrier. II. The effect of natural versus artificial feeding on intestinal permeability to macromolecules. *Paediatr Res* **1**(3): 245–9

UNAIDS (1999) Counselling and voluntary HIV testing for pregnant women in high HIV prevalence countries. Guidance for service providers (online). Available online: http://www.unaids.org/highband/document/mother-to-child/pisani.html (accessed 10 September, 1999)

Wemstron KD, Zuidema LJ (1989) Determination of opositive seoprevalence of HIV infection in gravidas by non anonymous screening. *Obstet Gynaecol* **74**: 558–61

Wilmington NC (2002) *The Antiretroviral Pregnancy Registry* (Interim Report) 1 Jan 1989–31 July 2000. Registry Project Office, London

Wimalasundera RC, Larbalestier N, Smith JH, de Ruiter A *et al* (2002) Pre-eclampsia, antiretroviral therapy, and immune reconstitution. *Lancet* **360**: 1152–4

World Health Organization (2004) HIV vaccine trial results are an important step forward in developing an effective vaccine, say WHO and UNAIDS (online). Available online: http://www.who.int/mediacentre/releases/2003/pr19/en/ (accessed 30 June, 2004)

Chapter 4

HIV screening during pregnancy: gender issues

The role of the midwife includes promoting health and providing health education to women and their families. The HIV epidemic is presenting midwives with fresh challenges in reducing the rate of heterosexual transmission of HIV, and in reducing the number of babies born with HIV as a result of vertical transmission. During the booking interview, midwives are required to offer and recommend HIV screening to all pregnant women (NHS Executive, 1999). This entails providing women with relevant information regarding HIV screening, and advising them in relation to 'safer sex' (Antenatal HIV Testing Working Party, 1998). This chapter examines the gender issues that arise when offering and recommending HIV screening to women during pregnancy. It also includes a discussion of the implications for midwifery practice.

Ensuring that women are aware of 'risk behaviour' may help to reverse the trend of women's increasing vulnerability to HIV. As there is a larger pool of infected men, women run a greater risk than heterosexual men of encountering an HIV-infected sexual partner, primarily in areas of high injection drug use and through sexual contact with a bisexual man (Campbell, 1995).

Studies have indicated that male-to-female transmission is significantly higher than female-to-male (Padian, 1987; Padian *et al*, 1987; Padian *et al*, 1991), because of a greater amount of HIV in semen as compared to vaginal and cervical secretions, and the greater amount of mucosal area exposed to HIV in the vagina. The vagina, acting as a receptacle, can be exposed for long periods of time. Adolescent girls are even more vulnerable because they have not yet developed mature mucosal defence systems. The cells lining the opening of the cervix are particularly susceptible to chlamydia, gonorrhoea and HIV (WHO, 2003).

Although women are more vulnerable, it has been argued that only targeting women to reduce the rate of heterosexual transmission is misguided, the reasons for this will be explored. This involves considering whether women are always aware of the risk behaviour of their partners, the ways in which traditional gender role socialisation discourages safer sex, gender power differences, and some difficulties faced by older women in long-term relationships in reducing risk behaviour.

Awareness of risk behaviour

Women may not always be aware of the past or present risk behaviour of their partners and, therefore, may not perceive themselves to be at risk. For example, male injecting drug users often secretly engage in this behaviour with other males, and even when female sex partners are aware of their partner's drug abuse, they may be unwilling to confront them for fear of physical violence or loss of economic support (Campbell, 1995).

Female sex partners may also be unaware of their risk because of the clandestine sexual behaviour of men who have sex with men and women. For example, one study which followed AIDS cases during 1981–1990, found that 25% of men who self-identified as bisexual were married when they died (Chu *et al*, 1992). Another study, which compared three groups of men who have sex with men and women, found that men who identified themselves as being gay, and those who identified themselves as heterosexual, practised safer sex with men, but not with women, whereas men who identified themselves as being bisexual practised safer sex with both men and women (Boulton *et al*, 1991). Some women may be both unaware of their partner's sexual behaviour and of the need to practice safer sex.

Traditional gender role socialisation

Prevention strategies that target women aim to get men to change their behaviour through women. Such strategies fail to acknowledge the following ways in which traditional gender role socialisation discourages safer sex:

⌘ Traditional male socialisation leads many men to believe that they must appear to know everything about sex, making it difficult for them to learn about HIV and safer sex from women (Campbell, 1995).
⌘ Male socialisation does not depict monogamy as an attractive way to demonstrate masculinity. The process of socialisation trains men to see sex as a conquest. The number of conquests they achieve is seen as an indicator of their manliness (Campbell, 1995).
⌘ Traditional socialisation portrays 'real men' as being heterosexual (Richardson, 1990; Wilton and Aggleton, 1991). It has been suggested that the lack of response to safer sex guidelines by heterosexual males may be their way of disassociating themselves from HIV because of homophobic fear (Campbell, 1995). Such fear leads men to deny that HIV has any relevance to them, and they continue to deny their own risk of infection and the risk that they may pose to their female partners.

According to Campbell (1995), the well-intentioned efforts of healthcare professionals to warn women about their risk takes pressure off men to practise safe behaviour, as whenever women are included as a specific target group, there is an implicit message that men are not. Although the attention to women's health is important, it perpetuates traditional beliefs about gender roles and serves to free men from taking responsibility for their own health and that of their female partners. For example, the specific targeting of women during pregnancy reinforces the belief that women are responsible for their own health and that of their children, a role which is frequently taken for granted in relation to HIV/AIDS (Du Guerny and Sjoberg, 1993). Targeting women undermines men's responsibility for the spread of HIV (Campbell, 1995). Society generally considers that it is the woman alone who is responsible for the contamination of her fetus (Bayer, 1989).

Gender power differences

Prevention strategies that target women fail to acknowledge gender power differences (Richardson, 1990; Ulin, 1992). For example, many women who are informed about the risk of unprotected sex are not in a position to use condoms because their male partners refuse to adopt such practice, as shown by The Women, Risk and AIDS Project (Holland *et al*, 1990a,b,c; 1991; 1992a,b; Thompson and Scott, 1991). The choices of safer sex for young women aged sixteen to twenty-one were constrained by the context of differential power relations in sexual encounters.

It has been argued that within the context of hetero-patriarchal discourse, constructs of sex are to do with penetration of a woman by a man, giving men the privilege of sexual pleasure, and constructing female subjectivity as powerless, pleasureless and androcentric. These gender inequalities mean that women have less power than men to control the progress and content of sexual interactions. Male needs and preferences predominate (Wilton and Aggleton, 1990).

One study, which looked at whether the same imbalance of power continues to affect older women's decisions, found that many women over the age of thirty still found it difficult to assert themselves in sexual relationships (Maxwell and Boyle, 1995). Most of the single women participating in the study used condoms in casual sexual relationships but this practice was often sporadic and short-lived. Most of them experienced difficulties in putting their wish to use condoms into practice because of men's attitudes, and although most of them felt strongly that the responsibility for 'safer sex' should be shared equally, they felt that they had to bear this responsibility on their own since men were reluctant to practice 'safer sex'.

Social and personal pressures

Even when women are able to challenge pressure from men to engage in unsafe sex, they are still susceptible to subtle personal and social pressures. For example, women comply with requests for sex because they do not wish to hurt their partner's feelings (Holland *et al*, 1992b). Also, peer group pressure can reinforce behaviour. When unsafe sex is the norm, people are more likely to practise unsafe sex rather than feel socially isolated or rejected (Maxwell and Boyle, 1995). In addition, the 'normalising social technologies of sex' (Gavey, 1992: 329) portrayed within the media and popular fiction provide models of sexual behaviour that can influence women. Such images often portray women's powerful ability to make men desire them, rather than a power that involves negotiating safer sex, and safer sex is rarely depicted.

Women in long-term relationships

It is often assumed that women in long-term relationships are not at risk. However, the British National Survey of Sexual Attitudes and Lifestyles found that 4.5% of married men and 1.9% of married women reported more than one sexual partner in the past year, rising to 16.6% and 9.3% respectively over a five-year period, and it is likely that there would be a further rise over a longer period. Among cohabiting couples, 15.3% of men and 8.2% of women reported more than one partner in the previous year, rising to 62% of men and 49.2% of women over a five-year period (Johnson *et al*, 1994). Monogamy in long-term relationships cannot be taken for granted.

The same survey also reported that only 21.8% of married women and 26.2% of cohabiting women used condoms for contraception, compared with 46.7% of single women. Maxwell and Boyle (1995) found that even when women knew their relationship had not been monogamous, or that their partner had previously been engaged in 'high-risk' behaviours, women only felt at risk if the relationship was casual. Condoms were generally discarded as soon as the relationship became established. The notion that a long-term relationship would automatically afford some magical protection was particularly striking. The most common reason for refraining from the use of condoms was trust. However, even when the trust was violated, women found difficulty in resuming safer sex. Difficulties in changing established behaviours were also experienced by women who had previously been using the pill when HIV was not an issue.

Patriarchal healthcare practices

Having considered these various gender issues, it would appear that although offering and recommending HIV testing to all pregnant women is clearly beneficial in terms of reducing the risk of vertical transmission, the opportunity for health promotion and subsequent HIV prevention is less certain, mainly because only women are targeted. Prevailing patriarchal forces within our society may have influenced the practice of targeting women when offering and recommending HIV testing during pregnancy.

Science and its application to reproduction was developed by men (Stacey, 1988), with the origins of modern medicine dating back to the scientific revolution of the seventeenth century. As such, the 'mechanistic model' formed a basis for the development of modern medicine, which has led to disease being defined primarily as a malfunctioning of one part of a mechanical body system, with little attention being paid to the prevention of illness, or emotional and social factors which affect health (Doyal and Elston, 1986).

This may explain why the focus of care provision is on the offer of a 'technological fix', for example recommending interventions to reduce the risk of MTCT, while HIV prevention and social issues, including gender inequalities, are virtually ignored. It is not surprising that modern medicine has been criticised for its failure to consider social factors in the causation of disease, and some believe the value of modern medicine should be examined, especially the way in which it can become a means of control, opposing or reinforcing wider social values (Doyal and Elston, 1986).

Feminists have argued that women's subordination occurs as a direct consequence of patriarchal healthcare practices, which result in women's needs being subordinated to men's (Nicolson and Ussher, 1992). While, there is evidence of wide acceptability of HIV screening among pregnant women, with the majority of women accepting out of consideration for the health of the unborn child (Larsson *et al*, 1990), the beneficial effects may be undermined if an unequal relationship exists between the doctor and the patient, or between the woman and the midwife. Such a relationship reinforces values and beliefs related to feelings of powerlessness that are common in different areas of life. With HIV testing during pregnancy, the doctor decides what the woman is suffering from and how it will be treated. This relationship fosters a belief that people have little control over their own bodies (Doyal and Elston, 1986).

It is important that midwives obtain informed consent (*Chapter 3*), thereby reducing potential harm when offering and recommending HIV testing during pregnancy. Although the woman prior to testing should give informed consent, their views about informed consent may be different from those of their health professionals. In one study, only 58.1% of women considered that they had given informed consent, although all health professionals felt that they had obtained it (Wieser *et al*, 1991). Midwives should reflect on their practice to ensure that women are enabled to act freely within the context of rational decision making (*Reader activity*).

Reader activity

❖ Reflect on your practice when offering antenatal HIV testing — identify a specific incident

❖ What information was given to enable the woman to choose whether to have the test?

❖ Was the information relevant and up-to-date?

❖ Was it sufficiently comprehensive, and presented in an appropriate way?

❖ Did the woman understand the information — how do you know?

❖ Were you aware of an unequal relationship between you and the woman?

❖ If so, how could this be addressed?

❖ Did you enable the woman to make a voluntary uncoerced decision?

❖ If not, what were the problems, and how might you change your practice in future, to enable a woman to be in control and act freely when choosing whether or not to have the test?

Society's response to HIV has challenged the democratic principals of human rights, and the corollaries of these principals, namely; tolerance, non-discrimination, protection of differences and individual's identities, which have guided legislative, health, social, educational and employment policies since the Second World War (Boltho-Massarelli, 1993). The main articles of the European Human Rights convention and European Social Charter relevant to public health (*Table 4.1*) provide a standard against which it is possible to judge the responses of all nations to HIV. Midwives, when offering and recommending HIV testing, should protect the right to liberty and security of a person by ensuring that a woman is not pressurised into having the test, or, any of the interventions, against her will. Midwives should also tackle discrimination where this occurs in practice, and reflect on their own behaviour to eradicate any form of discrimination.

HIV prevention efforts, which are caused by longstanding forms of societal discrimination towards people on the basis of their race or gender, have been identified as a major 'risk factor' for HIV prevention. Mann (1993: 3) writes, 'discrimination is a societal pathology which interferes with HIV prevention'. When targeting women during pregnancy, partner notification can be actively encouraged, giving contacts the opportunity to consider whether they wish to be tested (DoH, 1995). The injustice of expecting the woman to bear the full brunt of the emotional, psychological and social pressures associated with HIV testing cannot be ignored (Macquart-Moulin *et al*, 1995).

> ## Table 4.1: Main articles of the *European Human Rights Convention* and *European Social Charter* relevant to the public health field
>
> ❖   The right not to be subjected to inhuman or degrading treatment
>
> ❖   The right to liberty and security of person
>
> ❖   The right to marry and found a family
>
> ❖   The right to education
>
> ❖   The right to freedom of movement
>
> ❖   The right to protection of health
>
> ❖   The right to social security
>
> ❖   The right to social and medical assistance
>
> ❖   The right to benefit from social welfare services
>
> (cited by Boltho-Massarelli, 1993: 25)

Practice implications

The Chief Nursing Officer's review of the nursing, midwifery and health visiting contribution to vulnerable children and young people (DoH, 2004) recognises that midwifery care, delivered during pregnancy and the postnatal period, can determine long-term health outcomes for children. The review highlights a need for new extended roles for midwives who will specialise in public health. Several initiatives have been identified to enable midwives to further protect and promote the health of vulnerable children (*Table 4.2*).

This sphere of midwifery practice is seen as being 'hugely significant' and, when addressed, these initiatives will change the way in which some midwives will work. There will be more midwife consultants who will be responsible for public health and working with vulnerable families, such as those affected by HIV. An increasing involvement with fathers will mean greater opportunity for health promotion for vulnerable families in particular.

According to Campbell (1995), the upward trend in HIV infection rates among women will continue to rise until heterosexual men become the focus of prevention efforts, and HIV becomes conceptualised as a men's health issue. More attention needs to be paid to reproductive counselling for men, because, lowering the rate of infection among males has consequences both for women as sex partners and their future offspring. Mothers' concern about the future of their children acts as a primary motivation for them not to become infected with HIV (Population Reports, 1989; Sepulveda *et al*, 1992). HIV prevention strategies have incorporated themes about the need for mothers to stay healthy for their children. Prevention messages that promote the need for fathers likewise to stay healthy for their children, may also be beneficial.

Table 4.2: Future practice initiatives

❖ Continue to address workforce shortages

❖ Plan community midwifery services at a population level based on need

❖ Integration within children's centres and greater use of skill mix using maternity care assistants, will bring better continuity of care to vulnerable families from early pregnancy through to infancy. Families should experience a seamless and integrated midwifery and health visiting service. Continuity could be enhanced by the use of shared support workers and giving families a choice of practitioner

❖ Flexible on-going support following birth should be offered, rather than a chronologically determined cut-off point

❖ An increase in the number of new and extended roles for midwives, such as midwife consultants for public health, drug misuse and vulnerable families

❖ When midwives are located in children's centres they are more visible and accessible and able to identify vulnerable children early. Building on success of their role in Sure Start, consideration needs to be given to co-locating midwives in children's centres, while still being managed as a single service providing both community and hospital-based services

❖ Midwives need to work more effectively with fathers and be explicit in their responsibility for the child. While the value of woman-centred care is acknowledged, midwives need to assess the needs of the whole family, such as step-parents

❖ Additional training in child protection and in preparing and supporting vulnerable groups and families to become parents is needed

DoH, 2004

Research has shown that counselling and testing couples may have a beneficial effect on risk behaviour (Allen *et al*, 1992; Kamenga *et al*, 1991). Further research is required to assess the effectiveness of offering routine counselling and testing to couples during pregnancy as opposed to offering it to women only.

Improving human rights status and strengthening the dignity of people who are being discriminated against is also essential for the success of HIV prevention (Mann, 1993). Raising the status of women in society, particularly through self-empowerment and re-designing gender relations, are complementary strategies that should be adopted (Du Guerny and Sjoberg, 1993). Unless gender factors which influence the spread of HIV are addressed (*Table 4.3*), and goals are set to enable both partners to have equal influence over their sex lives (*Table 4.4*), the heterosexual spread of HIV is likely to continue rapidly (Du Guerny and Sjoberg, 1993).

Table 4.3: Gender factors which influence the spread of HIV

Society assigns men and women gender roles and unequal status

Women — lower status	Men — higher status
Lack of education/burden of housework and child care, caring for elderly and sick	Better chances for education/little or no responsibility for child care, housework or caring for elderly and sick
AIDS epidemic increases burden of traditional roles	
Lack of personal freedom/limited freedom of movement/limited access to information	Greater personal freedom/sexual freedom/ freedom of movement/access to information, including information on AIDS
Little or no control over family income and how it is spent	Wage income and control over it
Economic dependency	Power to make decisions
Little bargaining power in personal relations. Little influence over own and partner's sex life/inability to discuss sex with partner	Greater power to choose sexual partner/*de facto* right to have sexual partners, right to visit prostitutes/right to control sexual relationship with wife/partner

Overall outcome

Cannot demand safer sex	**Can choose whether to practice safer sex**

Areas to build on

Women's traditional roles make them good organisers	Can choose to change lifestyle and practice safer sex
Women have a tradition of organising self-help groups, that could be used to strengthen and empower women	Can choose to change attitude to women and actively to fight the epidemic

Obstacles to overcome

Dependency in certain areas	Machismo, expected to live up to the male ideal, which includes taking personal risks and endangering other's lives

Effect on HIV/AIDS epidemic

Power imbalance between gender roles facilitates the spread of the epidemic. By identifying the strong and weak points of each gender role, focal points for intervention may be identified.

(du Guerny and Sjoberg, 1993: 1029)

Table 4.4: Reducing heterosexual spread of HIV

Short-term goals

❖ Raising the status of women

❖ Focus on women's education and vocational training, to enhance women's economic independence

❖ Stressing the importance of gender-sensitive AIDS information to men and women

❖ Focus on community support to strengthen women's influence on, and control over, sexual relations

Long-term goals

❖ Programmes for changing attitudes to traditional gender roles, through tuition in schools, and other forms of public education

❖ Attempts to change stereotyped images of women and men in school books and mass media

❖ Reaching children and teenagers of both sexes early with information on AIDS and on protection from AIDS

❖ Reducing women's economic dependence through legal, economic and social measures, such as access to land, credit, child care and support to single mothers and female-headed households

❖ Promote, as a priority, the development of contraceptive and barrier methods which are effective against sexually transmitted diseases and AIDS, which correspond better to women's and men's needs

(du Guerny and Sjoberg, 1993: 1031)

Conclusion

In conclusion, reducing the spread of HIV by targeting pregnant women is inappropriate, ineffective, and can result in discrimination that interferes with HIV prevention. The focus on women is misguided because it assumes and gives women primary responsibility for safer sex practices. The effects of gender role socialisation and gendered power dimensions of heterosexuality cannot be ignored, as hetero-patriarchal constructs of sex affect women's risk behaviour.

In addition, patriarchal healthcare practices may contribute to women's oppression. For example, HIV screening of women may justify men's continued sexual behaviour, which puts women at risk. It may also reinforce a belief that women have little control over their own bodies.

The success of initiatives to educate women about their risk of HIV infection will depend on behavioural change of male partners. Therefore, priority must be given to a focus on men when implementing a health promotion strategy. Such strategies would have to be sensitive to the possibility of multiple and often clandestine sexual practices of heterosexual-identified men. In the same way that HIV prevention has targeted women in their role as mothers, men need to be targeted in their role as fathers. Research is required to assess the appropriateness of offering counselling and HIV testing to couples during pregnancy, as opposed to women only.

HIV prevention efforts should consider gender factors, such as raising the status of women and enabling both partners to have equal influence over their sex lives. From a global perspective, national policies need to ensure equal rights for women in relation to education, status and health care. Until the effects of gender inequalities are addressed within society, women will continue to be at risk of HIV. Future implications for midwifery practice include a greater role for consultant midwives in shaping public health and working with vulnerable families.

References

Allen S, Tice J, Van De Perre P *et al* (1992) Effect of serotesting with counselling on condom use and seroconversion among HIV serodiscordant couples in Africa. *Br Med J* **304**(6842): 1605–9

Antenatal HIV Testing Working Party (1998) *Quality framework for HIV testing services in London*. Inner London HIV Health Commissioners Group, London

Bayer R (1989) Perinatal Transmission of HIV Infection: The Ethics of Prevention. *Clin Obstet Gynaecol* **32**: 497–505

Boltho-Massarelli V (1993) *Transmissible Disease and Human Rights in Report of the 1993 Conference of European Community Parliamentarians on HIV/AIDS*. London International Group plc, London

Boulton M, Evans ZS, Fitzpatrick R, Graham H (1991) Bisexual men: women, safer sex and HIV transmission. In: Aggleton P, Hart G, Davies P, eds. *AIDS: Responses, Interventions and Care*. The Falmer Press, London: 65–78

Campbell CA (1995) Male gender roles and sexuality: implications for women's Aids risk and prevention. *Soc Sci Med* **41**(2): 197–210

Chu SY, Peterman TA, Doll S, Buehler JW, Curran JW (1992) AIDS in Bisexual Men in the United States: Epidemiology and Transmission to Women. *Am J Public Health* **82**(2): 220–5

Department of Health (1995) *The Health of the Nation Key Area Handbook. HIV/AIDS and Sexual Health*. DoH, London

Department of Health/User Experience and involvement/Professional
    Leadership Branch (2004) *The Chief Nursing Officer's review of the
    nursing, midwifery and health visiting contribution to vulnerable children
    and young people*. DoH, London
Doyal L, Elston MA (1986) Women health and medicine. In: Beechey V,
    Whitelegg E, eds. *Women in Britain Today*. Open University Press, Milton
    Keynes: 173–208
Du Guerny J, Sjoberg E (1993) Inter-relationship between gender relations
    and the HIV/AIDS epidemic: some possible considerations for policies
    and programmes. *AIDS* **7**(8): 1027–34
Gavey N (1992) Technologies and effects of heterosexual coercion. *Feminism
    and Psychology* **2**: 325–51
Holland J, Ramazanoglou C, Scott S (1990a) *WRAP Paper 1 — Sex, Risk and
    Danger: AIDS Education Policy and Young Women's Sexuality*. Tufnell
    Press, London
Holland J, Ramazanoglou C, Scott S, Sharpe S, Thompson R (1990b) Sex,
    Gender and Power: Young Women's Sexuality in the Shadow of AIDS.
    Sociol Health Illn **12**: 336–50
Holland J, Ramazanoglou C, Scott S, Sharpe S, Thompson R (1990c)
    *WRAP Paper 2 — 'Don't Die of Ignorance' — 'I Nearly Died of
    Embarrassment': Condoms in Context*. Tufnell Press, London
Holland J, Ramazanoglou C, Scott S, Sharpe S, Thompson R (1991) *WRAP
    Paper 6 — Pressure Resistance, Empowerment: Young Women and the
    Negotiation of Safer Sex*. Tufnell Press, London
Holland J, Ramazanoglou C, Scott S, Sharpe S, Thompson R (1992a) Risk,
    power and the possibility of pleasure: young women and safer sex. *AIDS
    Care* **4**: 273–283
Holland J, Ramazanoglou C, Sharpe S, Thompson R (1992b) *WRAP Paper
    7 — Pressured Pleasure: Young Women and the Negotiation of Sexual
    Boundaries*. Tufnell Press, London
Johnson AM, Wadsworth J, Wellings K, Field J (1994) *Sexual Attitudes and
    Lifestyles*. Blackwell Scientific Publications, Oxford
Kamenga M, Ryder R, Jingu M et al (1991) Evidence of marked sexual
    behaviour change associated with low HIV-1 seroconversion in 149
    married couples with discordant HIV-1 serostatus: experience at an HIV
    counselling centre in Zaire. *AIDS* **5**: 61–7
Larsson L, Spanberg L, Lindgren S, Bohlin AB (1990) Screening for HIV in
    pregnant women: a study of maternal opinion. *Aids Care* **2**(3): 223–8
Macquart-Moulin G, Hairion D, Auquier P, Manuel C (1995) Vertical
    transmission of HIV — a rediscussion of testing. *Aids Care* **17**(5): 657–62
Mann JM (1993) *AIDS Policy in Evolution: Learning From Experience
    Address, Report of the 1993 Conference of European Community
    Parliamentarians on HIV/AIDS*. London International Group plc, London
Maxwell C, Boyle M (1995) Risky heterosexual practices amongst women
    over 30: gender, power and long-term relationships. *AIDS Care* **7**(3):
    277–93

NHS Executive (1999) *Reducing mother to baby transmission of HIV. Health Service Circular 1999/183*. DoH, London

Nicolson P, Ussher J (1992) Introduction. In: Nicolson P, Ussher J, eds. *The Psychology of Women's Health Care*. Macmillan Press Ltd, London

Padian NS (1987) Heterosexual transmission of acquired immunodeficiency syndrome: international perspectives and national projections. *Rev Infectious Dis* **9**(5): 947–60

Padian NS, Marquis L, Francis DP *et al* (1987) Male-to-female transmission of human immunodeficiency virus. *J Am Med Assoc* **258**(6): 788–90

Padian NS, Shiboski SC, Jewell NP (1991) Female-to-male transmission of human immunodeficiency virus. *J Am Med Assoc* **266**(12): 1644–7

Population Reports (1989) AIDS education — a beginning. *Issues in World Health Series* L: 17–18

Richardson D (1990) AIDS education and women: sexual and reproductive issues. In: Aggleton P, Hart G and Davies P, eds. *AIDS: Individual, Cultural and Policy Dimensions*. The Falmer Press, London: 169–79

Sepulveda J Fineberg H, Mann J (eds) (1992) *AIDS Prevention Through Education: A World View*. Oxford University Press, Oxford

Stacey M (1988) *The Sociology of Health and Healing*. Unwin Hyman, London

Thompson R, Scott S (1991) *WRAP Paper 4 — Learning About Sex: Young Women and the Social Construction of Sexual Identity*. Tufnell Press, London

Ulin PR (1992) African women and AIDS: negotiating behavioural change. *Soc Sci Med* **34**(1): 63–73

Wieser S *et al* (1991) *Is voluntary HIV testing during pregnancy voluntary?* Proceedings of the Seventh International Conference on AIDS. Florence MC3333: 381

Wilton T, Aggleton P (1991) Condoms, coercion and control: heterosexuality and the limits to HIV/AIDS education. In: Aggleton P, Hart G, Davies P, eds. *AIDS: Responses, Interventions and Care*. The Falmer Press, London: 149–56

World Health Organization (2003) *Why are adolescents so vulnerable to sexually transmitted infections? Progress in Reproductive Health and Research*. Department of Reproductive Health and Research. WHO, Geneva

Chapter 5

The adoption of universal precautions in midwifery practice

Background

Prevention of occupational infection is an important issue for midwives when caring for women who may be unknowingly infected with HIV. 'Universal precautions' (UP) is now a common concept and guidelines have been developed to enable all healthcare workers to reduce their risk of occupational exposure to HIV, and other body fluid and blood-borne infections. However, issues surrounding implementation of UP into midwifery practice are complex. This chapter presents research undertaken by the author. The aim of the research is to assess and develop the practice of midwives in relation to the adoption of UP. Two focus group discussions were conducted with midwives who were practising within an inner London NHS trust, and a third was conducted with midwives who were practising in an NHS trust outside London. In addition, semi-structured interviews were conducted with the midwife managers from each of the two NHS trusts. The findings suggest that midwives do not always adequately protect themselves from occupational infection. The recommendations highlight the need for effective education, well-publicised guidelines and a conducive work environment to support good practice. Key midwives in the practice areas, acting as role models, appear to facilitate successful adoption of UP. As well as providing equipment, managers need to review the effectiveness of the equipment, and introduce safer devices as they become available.

Introduction

Midwives are increasingly at risk of exposure to HIV during the course of their work, particularly during delivery of the baby when there is an increased likelihood of exposure to blood and body fluids. Occupational exposure to HIV is particularly serious because there is no cure. In addition, there is a risk of occupational exposure to other blood-borne infections such as hepatitis B and hepatitis C.

There is no risk of infection being transmitted when blood from an HIV-infected patient comes into contact with a healthcare worker's intact skin. However, healthcare workers may become infected as a result of percutaneous exposure (PCE) to HIV-infected blood. This involves puncture of the skin by a needlestick, a sharp instrument, a human scratch or a bite (Health Protection Agency, 2004a). Recent figures suggest the risk is 0.31% (PHLS AIDS and STD Centre at the Communicable Disease Surveillance Centre and Collaborators, 1999). In other words, if 319 midwives sustained a needlestick injury, exposing themselves to HIV-infected blood, one of the midwives out of the 319 would become infected. Midwives can also become infected following mucotaneous exposure (MCE), defined as contamination of non-intact skin or mucous membranes (mouth, nose or eyes) (Health Protection Agency, 2004a). The risk from MCE is far lower, at about 0.03%. This equates to an HIV transmission risk of 1 in 3000 following contamination of mucous membranes, or, of broken skin, with infected blood or other infectious material, such as amniotic fluid or breast milk (PHLS AIDS and STD Centre at the Communicable Disease Surveillance Centre and Collaborators, 1999).

The transmission risk of HIV is less than the risk from an equivalent exposure to hepatitis B or hepatitis C virus. The transmission risk is about one in three for hepatitis B if the healthcare worker is unvaccinated, and around one in thirty for hepatitis C (PHLS AIDS and STD Centre at the Communicable Disease Surveillance Centre and Collaborators, 1999).

The concept of UP was first outlined in 1985 by the Centers for Disease Control (CDC, 1985). The CDC developed this concept and guidelines were issued to enable all healthcare workers to reduce their risk of occupational exposure to HIV, hepatitis B and hepatitis C (CDC, 1987; 1988; 1989). Current hospital guidelines and policies aim to reduce the risk of occupational exposure to body fluid and blood-borne infections through the use of UP. As it is not always possible to know whether people are infected, healthcare workers should regard all blood and body fluids as potentially infectious. The appropriate level of precautions to be taken for any procedure should be determined according to the extent of possible exposure and not because of knowledge of the patient's HIV status (DoH, 1998). Recommendations include taking precautions (*Box 5.1*), and staff are advised regarding vaccination against hepatitis B.

Since the introduction of routine screening for HIV during pregnancy, the HIV status of most women would be known at some point following testing. This may cause some midwives to question the need for UP when caring for women who are noted to be free from infection. However, the use of UP is still advisable as there is always a potential risk of infection. For example, some women may have contracted HIV since the initial blood test following unprotected sex with an infected partner. There is also a possibility that somebody may be sero-converting, and is therefore infected with HIV despite a negative test result. Furthermore, not all women agree to have the test, including some who know they are infected. They may choose to avoid disclosing their HIV status to their care providers, perhaps because they fear potential breaches of confidentiality and possible discrimination. The use of

UP is also recommended because of the need to protect against other infections which are not routinely screened for, such as hepatitis C.

However, the reality of adopting UP in midwifery practice is problematic and midwives do not always effectively minimise their risk of occupational exposure to infections through the adoption of UP. The potentially serious nature of the problem highlights the need for research to help close the theory/practice gap of midwives adopting UP. A qualitative research study was undertaken to explore the various complex issues surrounding the adoption of UP.

Box 5.1: Universal precautions

❖ Wearing gloves, masks, goggles, gowns and footwear when risk of exposure to body fluids, such as blood and amniotic fluid
❖ Safe disposal of sharp instruments
❖ Changing gloves between patients
❖ Washing hands when gloves are changed
❖ Appropriate disinfection of blood spillage/splashes
❖ Cover skin lesions
❖ Safe disposal of contaminated waste/linen/instruments

Research aim

The aim of the research was to assess and develop the practice of midwives in relation to adopting UP. The objectives were:

- to explore midwives' understanding of UP
- to examine the extent to which midwives are adopting UP in their practice
- to examine midwives' attitudes to UP
- to examine the factors which influence midwives' practice in relation to UP
- to explore ways of overcoming the problems identified
- to identify midwives' educational needs in relation to adopting UP.

Literature review

A literature search was undertaken using the Medline database. The search centred on the use of UP by healthcare workers and was restricted to publications from 1991–1996. The following themes were identified within the literature as being of relevance to the research problem:

- exposure mechanisms
- healthcare workers' compliance with UP
- factors which affect healthcare workers' compliance
- organisational factors related to successful implementation of UP in clinical practice.

Exposure mechanisms

Several of the studies (*Table 5.1*) reported that healthcare workers often fail to adequately protect themselves, as the recommendations for safe practice (*Box 5.1*) were not adhered to. Various exposure mechanisms were apparent (*Box 5.2*).

Failure to use appropriate barrier protection results in healthcare workers being exposed to potential infection. Almost 50% of the 541 American nurses in one study failed to use barrier protection when exposed to blood (Saghafi *et al*, 1992). Interestingly, when their hands were examined, just over half had acute or chronic skin lesions. Following implementation of UP, the rate of blood exposure to unprotected skin was far less. The protection afforded through wearing gloves when carrying out procedures which could result in exposure to blood or body fluid is clearly beneficial, particularly as it seems that healthcare workers often have tiny breaks in their skin. Failure to wear gowns when carrying out procedures where there is a likely risk of exposure to blood or body fluids to the arms and body has also been observed. Researchers, when conducting an observational study, found midwives' exposures to blood and amniotic fluid might have been prevented by the use of gowns (Panlilio *et al*, 1992). Another study of 306 American perinatal nurses showed that as barrier use by the nurses increased, their exposure to body fluid decreased (Bauer and Kenney, 1993).

However, some healthcare workers are exposed to infected blood and body fluids despite wearing barrier protection because of the poor quality of barrier protection available for staff. Bauer and Kenney (1993) identified barrier failures, such as; tearing gloves, gowns soaking through, leaking gloves and gloves that were too short, so that amniotic fluid went beyond the wrist when performing vaginal examinations.

Box 5.2: Exposure mechanisms

- ❖ Blood spashes to eyes (Kouri and Earnest, 1993)
- ❖ Hands — minor abrasions/eczema (Saghaffi *et al*, 1992)
- ❖ Gowns soaking (Bauer and Kenney, 1993)
- ❖ Gloves — tearing, leaking, too short (Bauer and Kenney, 1993)
- ❖ Re-sheathing needles (Schillo and Reischl, 1993; Henry *et al*, 1992)
- ❖ Sharps containers not changed regularly (Hersey and Martin, 1994)
- ❖ Needles left by bedside

Table 5.1: Studies relating to compliance with universal precautions

Researchers	Method	Sample
Bauer and Kenney (1993)	Questionnaire	306 American perinatal nurses
Hersey and Martin (1994)	Questionnaire	National survey — patient care staff
Schillo and Reischl (1993)	Questionnaire	1530 registered nurses in Michigan (random sample)
Roane (1993)	Observation	10 paediatric emergency room nurses (American)
Henry *et al* (1992)	Observation/ questionnaire	Healthcare workers in American hospital emergency department — low HIV prevalence area
Nelsing *et al* (1993)	Questionnaire	135 out of 168 nurses (80%) responded
Saghafi *et al* (1992)	Questionnaire	541 American nurses

Midwives are also at risk of blood splashes to the face when assisting with the delivery of a baby and when assisting during a caesarean section. Kouri and Ernest (1993) found that there was a substantial risk of blood or amniotic fluid splashes to the face during vaginal and caesarean deliveries. The obstetricians in the study all wore clear plastic face shields during fifty consecutive vaginal and fifty consecutive caesarean deliveries. The face shields were then examined for evidence of blood or amniotic fluid splashes. The researchers noted that 92% of the contaminated face shields were undetected by obstetricians at the time of caesarean delivery, and 50% were undetected at the time of the vaginal delivery. These results support the recommendation that midwives and obstetricians should wear protective eye glasses or face shields during all deliveries.

Another more serious risk of occupational infection is due to needle-stick injury. Saghafi *et al* (1992) found that the 541 nurses who completed a questionnaire sustained approximately two to eight needlestick injuries per nurse per year. According to the findings of a national survey, carried out in the United States of America, the most common reason for needlestick injury was re-sheathing needles (Hersey and Martin, 1994). Although, more than half of the PCEs reported by the 135 nurses who participated in a Danish study occurred without obvious explanation during medical procedures, or were caused by unexpected patient movement, a fifth of the nurses who sustained a PCE reported in a questionnaire that this occurred during disposal of an unshielded instrument (Nelsing *et al*, 1993). Re-sheathing a needle caused only one PCE, while a few nurses reported they sustained a PCE due to contact with an instrument temporarily left on a surface.

Compliance with universal precautions

Several studies have examined healthcare workers' compliance with UP. As shown in *Table 5.1*, most of these studies have used questionnaires. However, the use of questionnaires limits the reliability of the research findings because the honesty and accuracy of recall of the respondents cannot be guaranteed. To overcome this problem, other researchers have conducted observational studies. However, these also have limitations. For example, people may behave differently when they know that they are being observed. Healthcare workers who know they are being observed during a research trial may be more likely to wear barrier protection to be seen to be doing the right thing. The results could represent an underestimation of the problem. Roane (1993) attempted to overcome such biases by discarding data collected during the first hour of observation.

Despite these methodological criticisms, when looking at the findings overall, it appears that healthcare workers' compliance with UP is inadequate (see *Table 5.2*).

The study conducted by Hersey and Martin (1994) was a large national survey and there were a considerable number of non-respondents, which may have skewed the findings. However, the researchers conducted a pilot study and found that workers who responded only after being offered an incentive were similar in their compliance practices to workers who responded in the larger study. It could be assumed, therefore, that their research findings are reliable. They found inadequate compliance with wearing gloves, as shown by the fact that 64% of staff had reported blood on their hands during the preceding month. Compliance with wearing gowns, masks and goggles was poor, with only 24%, 19% and 10% wearing the respective attire.

Overall, from the findings recorded in *Table 5.2*, it appears that healthcare workers are more likely to wear gloves when appropriate, in comparison to the use of gowns, goggles and masks which were far less likely to be used when appropriate. One of the studies reported the use of two different methods. The researchers found no significant difference between self-reported glove use and re-sheathing of needles when observed and self-reported findings were compared (Henry *et al*, 1992). However, self-reported rates of other barrier use were significantly higher, compared with the observed rates of compliance. This suggests that the findings of the other studies, which relied on data obtained solely from questionnaires, represent an over-estimation of compliance in relation to gowns, masks and goggles.

Guidelines for good practice in safe disposal of sharps have been recommended (Wilson and Breedon, 1990):

- dispose of needles and other sharp instruments directly into a sharps container
- never re-sheath, bend or break needles
- discard needle and syringe as one unit into a sharps bin

- never fill sharps bins more than three-quarters full and ensure it is securely closed prior to disposal.

Table 5.2: Research findings in relation to compliance with universal precautions					
Researchers	**Disposal of needles**	**Use of gloves**	**Gowns**	**Masks**	**Goggles**
Nelsing *et al*		70%–100% depending on procedure			
Bauer and Kenney			Very poor	Very poor	Very poor
Hersey and Martin	Nearly half re-sheathed needles after taking blood. 96% always used sharps disposal containers	Inadequate. 64% reported blood/ body fluid on their hands at least once during the preceding month	Only 24% used	Only 19% used	Only 10% used
Schillo and Reischel	More than half re-sheathed needles. Nearly all used sharps disposable containers	More than 1/4 did not use gloves	Most had never used gowns		Most never used eye wear
Henry *et al*	Needles were re-sheathed 51% of the time. 5% of all needles were left unsheathed by the bedside or in the rubbish	Used 74% of the time	Used 12% of the time	Used 1% of the time	Used 13% of the time
Saghafi *et al*		46% had not used gloves			

The studies included in the literature review highlight some inconsistencies to these recommendations. For example, although the majority of healthcare workers in the studies correctly used sharps disposal containers, about half re-sheathed their needles (see *Table 5.2*). Furthermore, Hersey and Martin (1994) found that 38% of staff reported that sharps containers had been full 'sometimes' or 'often' in the last month, and some had sustained a sharps injury due to a sharp sticking out of the sharps disposal container.

Factors affecting compliance

The studies which examined factors affecting healthcare workers' compliance with UP are identified in *Table 5.3*.

Table 5.3: Studies relating to factors which affect compliance	
Researchers	**Method**
Bauer and Kenney (1993)	Questionnaire
Saghafi *et al* (1992)	Questionnaire
Schillo and Reischl (1993)	Questionnaire
Gershon *et al* (1995)	Questionnaire — confidential survey of 1716 hospital-based healthcare workers from three geographically distinct populations
Henry *et al* (1992)	Observation/questionnaire
Nelsing *et al* (1993)	70–100% depending on the procedure

Research undertaken by Gershon *et al* (1995) showed that although most of the 1,716 workers who returned their questionnaires were extremely knowledgeable about UP, this knowledge was not necessarily associated with compliance. Various factors appear to motivate staff to adopt UP (see *Table 5.4*). Factors that appear to make staff less likely to use UP have been identified in *Table 5.5*.

Table 5.4: Motivational factors

❖ Perception that all patients are potentially infectious (Bauer and Kenney, 1993)

❖ Fear of occupational transmission of HIV (Gershon *et al*, 1995)

❖ Working in high infection prevalence area (Gershon *et al*, 1995)

❖ Perception that adoption of UP lowers risk of occupational infection (Gershon *et al*, 1995)

❖ Tolerant attitude towards HIV/AIDS patients (Gershon *et al*, 1995)

❖ Training — highest compliance associated with six or more hours each year (Gershon *et al*, 1995)

❖ Perception that hospital has a strong commitment to safety standards (Gershon *et al*, 1995)

Table 5.5: Barriers to the use of universal precautions

❖ Not enough time in an emergency (Bauer and Kenney, 1993; Schillo and Reischl, 1993)

❖ Poorly fitting gloves/gowns (Bauer and Kenney, 1993; Schillo and Reischl, 1993)

❖ Gloves/gowns leak (Bauer and Kenney, 1993)

❖ Glove material causes allergic dermatitis (Bauer and Kenney, 1993)

❖ Lack of availability of barrier protection (Bauer and Kenney, 1993; Schillo and Reischl, 1993)

❖ Poor managerial commitment to UP (Bauer and Kenney, 1993; Gershon *et al*, 1995)

❖ Vaccinated against hepatitis B (Bauer and Kenney, 1993)

❖ Used good hand washing (Bauer and Kenney, 1993)

❖ Patient 'low risk' (Bauer and Kenney, 1993; Saghafi *et al*, 1992)

❖ Gloves interfere with ability to perform procedures (Bauer and Kenney, 1993; Saghafi *et al*, 1992; Gershon *et al*, 1995; Schillo and Reischl, 1993)

❖ Barrier protection awkward/poorly constructed (Schillo and Reischl, 1993)

❖ Risk-taking personality (Gershon *et al*, 1995)

❖ High levels of work stress (Gershon *et al*, 1995)

Two of the studies have clearly shown that many staff, particularly those working in a low HIV prevalence area, attempt to determine whether or not the patient is in a 'high risk' category and adopt infection control measures accordingly (Bauer and Kenney, 1993; Henry *et al*, 1992). Henry *et al* (1992), who conducted their research in a low HIV prevalence area, reported that higher rates of glove or gown use were observed during interactions with males and non-whites who tended to be young. Fifty per cent of the healthcare workers indicated that patient appearance affected their decisions regarding compliance with UP. The findings from both the observed and self-reported data indicate that healthcare workers attempt to determine which patients are likely to be infected and exercise discriminate caution.

The literature has identified a wide range of factors that affect whether or not healthcare workers adopt UP in their practice. These include personal factors, such as: the risk-taking personality of individual practitioners; factors associated with the client population, such as the prevalence of HIV; managerial commitment to implementing a UP policy, including provision of comfortable and appropriate barrier protection that is easily accessible in the work area; and provision of continuing training to enable staff to adopt UP in practice.

Organisational factors

Several of the researchers have made suggestions in relation to creating an 'organisational climate' which may help foster the use of UP in practice.

The suggestions (*Table 5.6*) illustrate how effective implementation of a UP policy requires a high degree of commitment from managers. Such commitment involves action, ranging from raising awareness through simple measures such as putting posters in strategic locations, through to facilitating forums where staff can raise issues. These forums enable problems such as workplace stress and equipment availability and adequacy to be discussed and managed. Managers need to identify ways of targeting individual members of staff where particular problems have been identified and recommending appropriate interventions, such as further training.

Suggestions for staff training have been summarised in *Table 5.7*. Gershon *et al* (1994) facilitated focus group discussions which enabled them to provide further suggestions for making the training more effective. Various teaching methods, such as role-play and simulations, would be appropriate for effectively implementing their suggestions. In addition, educators could facilitate midwives to reflect on their practice and analyse the issues. Skilled educators are essential for the delivery of high quality education and training to ensure effective outcomes.

Table 5.6: Facilitating a conducive 'organisational climate'
❖ Display posters in work areas (Hersey and Martin, 1994)
❖ Assess staff compliance during individual performance review (IPR) (Hersey and Martin, 1994)
❖ Ensure staff adhere to hepatitis B vaccination programme (Hersey and Martin, 1994)
❖ Examine work practices to reduce PCE (Hersey and Martin, 1994)
❖ Availability/accessibility/comfort of protective barrier precautions and equipment (Hersey and Martin, 1994)
❖ Strategic location of sharps disposal containers (Hersey and Martin, 1994)
❖ Ensure sharps containers emptied regularly (Hersey and Martin, 1994)
❖ Managers to evaluate quality/adequacy of barrier protection provided (Bauer and Kenney, 1993)
❖ Supervisory support and counselling for workers who demonstrate risk-taking personalities (Gershon *et al*, 1995)
❖ Limiting workplace stress (Gershon *et al*, 1995)

Table 5.7: Suggestions for effective training
❖ Staff to receive initial and continuing training (Gershon *et al*, 1994; Hersey and Martin, 1994; Saghafi *et al*, 1992)
❖ Interactive training sessions to allow workers to become more familiar with the use of UP in emergency situations (Gershon *et al*, 1994)
❖ Should address workers' perception of risk (Gershon *et al*, 1994)
❖ Should address situations where workers experience conflict between the need to protect themselves and the need to provide patient care (Gershon *et al*, 1994)

Research methodology

Rationale for research methodology

Qualitative research was undertaken to assess and develop the practice of midwives in adopting UP. The majority of studies in the literature review used questionnaires for data collection, which limited the exploration of factors influencing the use and non-use of UP. Focus group discussions were used in this study to examine whether the same factors influence midwives' practice, and to provide a more in-depth analysis of the research problem. The rationale for the chosen methodology is that the intense involvement between the researcher and the research participants, and the probe for the most truthful responses, yields a more in-depth analysis with focus group discussions compared to that produced by quantitative methods (Mariampolski, 1984).

Triangulation was employed to enhance the validity of the research. This involved collecting data through the use of two methods, and examining differing perspectives. Focus group discussions provided the means to explore midwives' understanding of and attitudes to UP, to examine the extent to which UP were being adopted and to examine the factors which influenced the adoption of UP by midwives. In addition, semi-structured interviews enabled further exploration of the adoption of UP by midwives from a managerial perspective. A midwife manager from each of the two hospitals selected for the focus group discussions was interviewed. An outline of the interview schedule is displayed in *Table 5.8*.

Table 5.8: Semi-structured interview of clinical midwife manager

1	Has the introduction of UP presented any particular issues for you as a manager?
2	Do you feel satisfied with the way midwives are adopting UP?
3	What do you consider to have worked successfully in relation to implementing the adoption of UP by midwives?
4	What are the problems you have encountered? ie. staff attitude, policy, equipment, costs, reporting of accidental injuries.
5	What arrangements do you have for staff development and education?

The methodology of focus groups and the importance of interaction of research participants has been explored by Kitzinger, who describes focus groups as, 'group discussions organised to explore a specific set of issues' (1994: 103). Dimensions of understanding may be revealed that often remain untapped by the more conventional one-to-one interview or questionnaire. Discussion with others who share similar experiences encourages participants to express, clarify and develop particular perspectives. Differences of opinion can be explored as participants are encouraged to explain the reasoning behind their thinking (Kitzinger, 1994).

Focus groups, typically, have high face validity, due to the credibility of comments from the participants (Nyamathi and Shuler, 1990). They can generate more critical comments than interviews (Watts and Ebbutt, 1987), and they encourage participation from midwives who may be reluctant to be interviewed on their own. The inter-personal communication can also highlight (sub) cultural values or group norms (Kitzinger, 1995). The group provides mutual support when feelings are expressed which are common to their group but which they might consider deviant from mainstream culture, or the assumed culture of the researcher (Kitzinger, 1994). Through analysing the humour, consensus, dissent and different types of narratives used within the group, shared and common knowledge may be identified (Hughes and Dumont, 1993).

Ethnographers have argued that meanings and interpretations are not fixed entities (Atkinson, 1979). They are generated through social interaction and it is possible that they may change over the course of such interaction. Midwives are not isolated, static entities, and their personal behaviour is not cut off from public discourses. They are part of complex and overlapping social, familial and collegiate networks. Therefore, it makes sense to use research methods that actively encourage the examination of these social processes in action (Kitzinger, 1994). Midwives' identities are subject to processes of 'becoming', rather than being fixed and static as they adopt the practice of UP. During periods of change midwives may need to question their beliefs. Focus group discussions provide the means to clarify issues, to consider ways of developing practice, and to consider educational and developmental needs.

Ethical issues

A research proposal was submitted to the Healthcare Nursing Research/Ethics Committee of the inner London hospital and, in accordance with hospital policy, approval was sought before proceeding with the research. Consent was obtained from the heads of midwifery services to undertake the research in both of the hospitals, including written consent from the head of midwifery services of the inner London hospital, as required by their Healthcare Nursing Research/Ethics Committee. The midwifery managers from both hospitals enabled me to approach midwives who would be available to participate in the focus group discussions. Each of the midwives was given a letter, explaining the purpose of the research, and those who agreed to participate were asked to sign a consent form. The two midwifery managers were also given an explanatory letter and asked to sign a consent form. Written permission was also sought from the head of midwifery services of another midwifery unit to take photographs for the purpose of the research, while ensuring that no individuals were identifiable.

Sample selection

Convenience samples of midwives participated in the focus group discussions. Although random selection would reduce bias, it is not the primary factor in the selection of focus group participants (Kreuger, 1994). The reality of the workplace dictated the selection, as the managers had to balance the needs of the service with the research requirements, and workload constraints affected the size of the samples. It is possible that the voluntary nature of the selection may have resulted in the inclusion of midwives who were more highly motivated about adopting UP. The selection of participants was restricted to practising midwives as superior or subordinate relationships among participants may inhibit the discussion (Kreuger, 1994). This is known as a homogenous group. The inclusion of women or 'service users', midwife managers, an HIV counsellor or an infection control nurse may have affected the degree of self-disclosure by the midwives.

However good the arrangements are, Kreuger (1994) points out that researchers should always be ready for the unexpected. One of the unpredictable elements in my research was the small number of midwives who were available to participate in the discussion groups. Although I had planned for the groups to consist of approximately eight midwives, on the actual day only six midwives took part in the first group, and four took part in the second group within the inner London hospital. The third group consisted of only three midwives within the hospital outside London. Kreuger (1994) states that if only a few people attend for the focus group discussion, the session should be carried out as planned.

The importance of providing incentives has been highlighted in the literature (Kreuger, 1994). Tea, coffee and currant buns were provided for the midwives as they arrived prior to the discussion sessions, which were conducted in a convenient location within the maternity unit. The discussion time was restricted to one hour, which was a realistic time commitment for the participants.

Focus groups discussions

Three focus groups discussions were facilitated in October 1996. Undertaking two in an inner London hospital, and a third in a hospital outside London, enabled a comparison to be made of midwives' attitudes and practice between the two hospitals. Outside London the number of HIV-infected women attending antenatal clinics was considerably lower, compared to rates in inner London (*Figure 3.1, p.38*). The midwives working in inner London were offering women routine screening for HIV during pregnancy, and many had undergone training for this role. The preparatory study day included a session on the use of UP to protect against occupational HIV infection. In contrast, the hospital outside London did not have a routine HIV screening policy for pregnant women at the time the study was undertaken.

A questionnaire was devised with the intention of using it prior to the focus groups to trigger some discussion. It was piloted with a group of midwives who were attending an HIV study day for midwives practising in the inner London hospital. However, this yielded limited data, and so scenarios (opposite) and photographs were used instead. To achieve consistency, a format for the focus group discussions was developed. This was tested with a group of student midwives during a teaching session and refined slightly (*Box 5.3*).

According to Nyamathi and Shuler, 'the hallmark for the focus group is the quality in which spontaneity and candour is obtained' (1990: 1283). Passive participants may be influenced or inhibited by other more vocal participants, and respondents have a tendency to be polite and fit in with the group norm by complying (McQuarrie and McIntyre, 1987). Therefore, attention was given to creating an environment that would encourage all participants to divulge emotions that often remain untapped. During the introduction, I emphasised that there are no right or wrong answers, but rather differing points of view, and that I was interested in hearing each person's views. I encouraged participants to share negative and positive thoughts and feelings. The opening question required each member to introduce herself, providing an 'ice breaker'.

As the discussion progressed the questions became more focused. The research process is dynamic, and skilful probing enables questions to be asked and nourished (Kreuger, 1994). Participants often form opinions or change and develop their views as they hear or are challenged by the perspectives of others. Views were clarified during the discussions, and the questioning was adjusted to capitalise fully on the discussion as it evolved.

Scenarios

Scenario 1: You have taken a sample of blood from a lady who has given a history of having a partner who has been an intravenous drug user. Inadvertently, you sustain a needlestick injury. How would you react? What would you do?

Scenario 2: You are taking a sample of blood from a professional Caucasian lady following a booking interview. Inadvertently you sustain a needlestick injury. How would you react? What would you do?

Scenario 3: You are clearing up after a forceps delivery. As there was a postpartum haemorrhage, there is quite a large amount of blood spillage. How would you deal with cleaning the bed, floor and trolley, and the disposal of bloodstained instruments, sharps and rubbish?

Scenario 4: You are required to take a routine newborn blood spot screening test on a baby who has been transferred home. What precautions would you take to reduce your risk of blood-borne infection?

Scenario 5: You have attended a home birth. What precautions would you take when examining and disposing of the placenta to reduce the risk of blood-borne infection? How would you reduce your risk of needlestick injury?

The quality of the research is determined by the way in which the asking, listening, understanding and re-telling is done. I used open-ended questions to avoid 'subtle topic control', and consistently adopted the stance of a learner (May, 1991). Webb believes that the researcher's 'personal beliefs and values enter the process throughout' (1992: 748). To reduce the possibility of influencing the responses, I tried to adopt a neutral stance and adjusted my body language accordingly. Also, when necessary, I summarised some of the information during the discussion by reflecting back to the group what I felt they were saying, to verify that this was a correct assessment of the issues being discussed.

For the purpose of data collection, the focus group discussions and interviews were audio-taped. At a certain point theoretical saturation is reached, when nothing new emerges from the data. Kreuger (1994) suggests that following three focus group discussions, there is usually little need to proceed further as no new findings appear.

Role of assistant moderator

I arranged for a colleague, who was also a senior lecturer in midwifery, to take on the role of assistant moderator. This entailed turning the tape over, and noting key points, pertinent quotations, body language and cues, such as silences or giggles (Kreuger, 1994). Following the discussion we tape-recorded our 'de-briefing' which formed part of the research data.

Box 5.3: Format for focus group discussions

Introduction: Highlight commonality of group members — all are practising midwives selected because I am interested in hearing your views on UP in midwifery practice.

Opening question:

Can you introduce yourself and state what area you work in? (name cards were displayed in front of each participant)

Introductory questions:

What do you think of UP?

❖ Use scenarios to stimulate discussion in relation to practice.

Transition questions:

❖ Do you think UP necessary?

❖ What has enabled you to develop an understanding of UP?

Key questions:

1. Drawing on your experiences, to what extent do you feel the use of UP is practical?

2. What prompted you to adopt UP?

3.* What aspects of UP do you feel particularly at ease with?

4.* What aspects do you have problems with?

* Photographs were used to provide cues

After looking at these photographs, are there any additional needs/feelings/views that come to mind?

Sentence completion:

7. Now, as I think about the adoption of UP, what really helped me was...

Each participant was encouraged to write down their thoughts and share it with the group.

Ending questions:

❖ Summary question: moderator to summarise key ideas that emerged from the discussion (2–3 minutes)

Ask group if this is an adequate summary.

❖ Final question: allow 10 minutes. Purpose of discussion was to examine midwives' feelings/understanding and needs in relation to the use of UP. Have we missed anything?

Analysing the results

The main goal of gathering data from the focus group discussions is to generate detailed narrative data (Knafl and Howard, 1984), which enables a systematic study of the world of everyday experience to be achieved (Nyamathi and Shuler, 1990). The process of systematically analysing the data began with playing back the tape recordings and making detailed word processed notes, comparing the responses to each of the questions. The same process was followed for the semi-structured interviews. Key quotations, which captured the feelings of the midwives were included in the analysis, and themes or patterns were identified. The use of verbatim quotes provides verification of the authenticity of the findings (Polit and Hungler, 1998).

Hisrich and Peters (1982) have defined a theme as being a concept expressed in one or more terms. Minority views should also be included in the analysis. When participants express differing views, the absence of patterns in the data can be a meaningful discovery (Kreuger, 1994).

Kreuger (1994) believes that the analysis should seek to provide enlightenment, and that understanding should be lifted to a new plateau. This involves asking the following questions:

1 What was known and then confirmed or challenged by this study?
2 What was suspected and then confirmed or challenged by this study?
3 What was new that wasn't previously suspected?

Another strategy involves comparing and contrasting the results with established theory in social science. Diagrams may also be used to provide visual, symbolic images that can demonstrate links to enhance critical understanding.

The analytical process should permit another researcher to arrive at similar conclusions using available documents and raw data. As Kreuger (1994) points out, there may be a tendency to see or hear selectively only those comments which confirm a particular viewpoint, while omitting information that causes researcher dissonance. Verification in analysis is a critical safeguard. For this to occur there must be sufficient data to constitute a trail of evidence (Kreuger, 1994). The raw data consisted of the tape recordings of the focus group discussions, the de-briefing with the assistant moderator and the semi-structured interviews, as well as the assistant moderator's notes. The word-processed transcripts comparing the responses to the questions formed part of the 'audit trail', providing an accurate record of the various stages of data collection and data analysis (Holloway and Wheeler, 1996).

Results

The results are presented according to the themes identified (see *Table 5.9*).

Table 5.9: Research themes
❖ The extent to which midwives use barrier protection
❖ Practice issues related to risk reduction
❖ Areas of ambiguity
❖ Fear of infection
❖ Evidence of discriminatory practice
❖ Barriers to the adoption of UP
❖ Factors which motivated midwives to adopt UP
❖ Managerial issues

The extent to which midwives use barrier protection

Although the midwives generally recognised the need to adopt UP in practice, they did not always adequately protect themselves from blood and body fluids. Some variation was found in relation to the extent of the precautions that were adopted, particularly when comparing the practice of the midwives in inner London with those outside London.

Gloves/gauntlets

All of the midwives wore gloves when assisting women who were giving birth. Also, the midwives from inner London wore gauntlets when assisting women who chose to give birth in water. For other procedures where exposure to blood or body fluids was likely, the midwives in inner London generally wore gloves, although some inconsistencies were apparent, for example, when poorly fitting gloves interfered with their ability to take blood. Also, one midwife said she did not always use gloves for changing inco-pads. However, the midwives outside London were not in favour of wearing gloves when obtaining a blood sample from a woman or from a baby's heel, even if the gloves were close fitting.

Gowns/plastic aprons

The midwives from inner London normally wore gowns when assisting women who were giving birth. However, the midwives outside London said they normally evaluated each case before determining the extent of the precautions they would adopt, and they would not normally wear gowns. One midwife implied that wearing a plastic apron was more 'practical', stating, 'it's easy to put gloves and a pinny on for a delivery'.

Eye protection

The midwives from inner London were all familiar with the need to wear goggles when assisting women who were giving birth, although one midwife preferred to wear glasses rather than goggles. However, none of the midwives from outside London used goggles.

Masks

There was general consensus that masks and plastic visors did not need to be worn during deliveries.

Protective footwear

The inner London midwives tended to wear protective footwear when exposure to blood was likely. Plastic overshoes were usually worn, although one midwife said she kept a pair of shoes specifically for wearing on the delivery suite. The midwives outside London thought it was unnecessary to wear protective footwear, unless they were working in theatre.

Practice issues related to risk reduction

Various practice issues were discussed in relation to reducing the risk of exposure. Ways of reducing risk of exposure were identified, sometimes, as an alternative to using the recommended barrier protection. For ease of presentation, these have been categorised under the following sub-headings.

Disposal of placenta

There was considerable discussion regarding the need to reduce blood spillage when disposing of the placenta. Although different ways of wrapping placentas were discussed, there seemed to be some agreement that this was best achieved by wrapping the placenta securely in a paper towel and then wrapping it in a yellow bag which was secured, before placing it in another yellow bag for incineration. When conducting a home delivery, the midwives from outside London also said that ice cream containers could be used for transporting the wrapped placenta to hospital.

Clearing up after a delivery

Generally, all midwives recognised the need to protect their hands from blood, and would therefore wear gloves when handling bloodstained linen and instruments. One midwife said that if there was a lot of blood spillage following a delivery, she would always use gloves and a plastic apron when clearing up.

Newborn blood spot screening

The midwives identified various risk reduction strategies to obtaining blood for newborn blood spot screening. Although gloves were not always worn, one midwife outside London referred to hand washing. The inner London midwives talked about laying the baby down, or getting the mother to hold the baby, securing the legs, 'because when the baby kicks, the blood goes all over the place'. They also noted that the card was sometimes placed in the envelope with the blood spots exposed. Suggestions for good practice included writing the baby's details on the card before obtaining the blood sample, and placing the package within a sealed specimen bag.

Venepuncture

There was some agreement that the use of vacutainers would reduce the risk of occupational infection compared with using a needle and syringe for taking blood. However, not all the midwives used vacutainers. One midwife from outside London said, 'I've not seen them before', and another said she used vacutainers but found them 'such a fiddle'.

One midwife from inner London said she had never been shown how to use a vacutainer. She argued from a personal perspective that using a syringe was less painful for the patient, stating, 'I'm never going to inflict that pain on someone, so I don't use them'.

Disposal of needles and sharp instruments

The following areas of 'good practice' in the safe disposal of needles and sharp instruments were identified:

1 Needles should not be removed from syringes.
2 Excess thread should be cut from suture needles.
3 Needles should be counted.
4 Doctors should be asked to clear their own trolleys, to avoid hazards from any loose needles that may be covered by the used gown.
5 Sharps bins should be located in each room.
6 Sharps disposal containers should not be left to become over full — this was seen as everybody's responsibility.
7 Needles should not be re-sheathed.

Hepatitis B vaccination

One midwife pointed out the need to ensure that hepatitis B vaccinations were up to date.

Perineal suturing

The manager in inner London advocated suturing tears only where necessary, maintaining that some second-degree tears do not require suturing, unless bleeding. One of the midwives from inner London referred to a study that was being conducted to assess the benefits of leaving second-degree perineal tears unsutured. The midwives also pointed out the importance of suturing technique, such as using forceps to hold the needle, rather than using their fingers. One midwife said she wore two pairs of gloves, 'just to make absolutely sure'.

Blood splashes to the eyes

The inner London midwives discussed how they could reduce the incidence of blood splashes to the eyes, for example, one midwife mentioned 'milking the cord'. They also discussed eye protection, and agreed that glasses were more practical than goggles, although they felt more protected wearing goggles.

Protective footwear

The midwives tended to decide whether the wearing of protective footwear was necessary based upon the degree of blood loss expected. Most of the midwives, apart from some practising in inner London, preferred not to wear protective footwear during normal deliveries. One midwife commented, 'I try to keep my legs away from the blood'. However, one of the midwives from inner London argued that overshoes or plastic boots should be worn during instrumental deliveries in view of the increased risk of blood spillage. Wellingtons were available for doctors' use during instrumental deliveries, and they were required to clean their own wellingtons with 'Hibiscrub'.

Masks

According to the manager in inner London, the wearing of masks during normal deliveries was unnecessary, provided 'good technique' was used, ie. covering the cord before cutting it.

Water births

It was felt that the bath should be washed with chlorhexidine solution following a water birth.

Informing women

The inner London midwives felt that most couples understood why UP were being implemented, and that explanations regarding the use of UP should ideally be given to the woman and her partner before delivery, if time permitted. They pointed out that for women who were admitted late in labour and 'pushing' this might be difficult. One midwife laughed, saying, 'she couldn't care less really' what the midwives were wearing!

Areas of ambiguity

Several areas of ambiguity and confusion were apparent.

Disposal of blood-stained linen

One midwife from inner London commented that although bloodstained linen should be disposed of in double bags, ie. a plastic inner bag surrounded by a red nylon outer bag, it tended to be placed in clear plastic bags, together with non-blood-stained linen. This was because bloodstained linen was rarely seen on the ante/postnatal ward, and it seemed easier just to use the one bag.

Protective footwear

Some discrepancy was also noted among the inner London midwives about wearing protective footwear when assisting women to deliver their babies, as reflected in the following comment: 'we are supposed to, but we don't always get to'.

Disposal of placenta

The inner London midwives were also concerned that the hospital porters were sometimes exposed to risk of infection due to the failure of some midwives to dispose of the placentas safely. They said that the hospital porter transported the placentas in a bucket, and that they (the midwives) should seal the lid securely with tape to prevent the placentas from falling out in transit, but this did not always happen. In addition, instead of wrapping the placentas, some midwives just threw them into the bucket, which was lined with a plastic bag, 'one on top of the other'. They noted that the bags were not very strong and could split easily because, as one midwife asked, 'how many placentas can a bucket hold?' One midwife said she saw blood all over the floor, which was 'not very nice for the porters if the midwives hadn't wrapped it properly'. They acknowledged the need to ensure other staff were not put at risk through their negligence, and that they could be liable, 'because we are the ones who disposed of this potentially dangerous item.'

Cleaning instruments

Some of the inner London midwives washed instruments to remove any blood before sending them to be autoclaved, whereas others did not. One midwife commented, 'you put yourself more at risk by washing them'. However, another said, 'it's nicer for someone else if you've washed them'. She also said that she had seen instruments returned from CSSD with congealed blood attached to the grooves of forceps, which justified the practice of washing them.

Cleaning blood spillages/splashes

The inner London midwives expressed uncertainty regarding whether granules should be used for cleaning blood spillages, and how long the granules should be left on the spillage to destroy effectively any infection. In addition, inconsistencies were apparent in cleaning blood splashes on beds and trolleys. After some discussion, the midwives in one group agreed that chlorhexidine-based soap was used. Most of the midwives in the second group said the trolleys were cleaned with soap and water and sprayed with 'hycholin' spray, while one said she cleaned the blood off with cold water prior to using 'hycholin' spray. One midwife commented that she had been told not to use hyperchloride solution for cleaning blood splashes on plastic mattress covers, as it may ruin the plastic.

The midwives outside London used 'Precept' for cleaning blood splashes. However, when shown the photographs later in the discussion they said that 'Actichlor' tablets dissolved in water were used.

Needlestick injury

There appeared to be some confusion among one group of inner London midwives regarding whether to squeeze the puncture wound following a needlestick injury. One midwife said the occupational health sister told her not to squeeze the affected finger as 'you do not know what is around the site and you may be forcing things in, as opposed to letting whatever is around the site come out if it was just allowed to bleed freely'. Other midwives were unaware of this advice, and so they wanted clarification.

In addition, the inner London midwives appeared to be uncertain about obtaining consent for HIV testing of the source patient following needlestick injury. One of the midwives said she would explain to the lady that, 'for it to be safe, we have to take some blood from you and store it... just in case'. Another midwife said, 'you should really tell her that you are doing it... this should be done in a tactful way so that she doesn't get too upset about it... because she might be thinking — "oh, so you think I've got HIV or something" '.

The manager from the hospital outside London was unsure about whether the source patient would be offered pre-test counselling, and who should provide this for the affected midwife as well as the source patient.

Isolation

The midwives outside London spoke about reducing the flow of people in and out of the room of an HIV-infected woman as they felt this would provide some protection for other members of staff. This practice appears to be ambiguous, and was not supported by a clear rationale.

Disposal of needles and sharp instruments

Although there was general agreement regarding 'good practice' related to safe disposal of needles and sharp instruments, some inconsistency was noted. For example, one midwife said she still saw midwives re-sheathing needles, because it was a 'habit'. Another midwife, from outside London said,

> *I always re-sheathe my needles... I'd rather do that than leave... like if you've got a little tray with all your bits and pieces, then I think you could easily pick it up and cut your finger on the end of it. So I know we're not meant to, but I always do.*

Fear of infection

Some of the midwives from inner London expressed considerable fear of the possibility of becoming infected following a needlestick injury. Their comments included feeling 'threatened', 'frightened', 'shock' and 'panic'. One midwife said, 'everything would go through my mind, Oh God!' Another said 'do I really want to have my blood taken, just to check? — what would be the consequences if I had this test done to tell me what I do not want to know?'

However, some of the midwives laughed and seemed to perceive their risk following a needlestick injury as being quite low. One midwife commented, 'you could just wash your hands without making a fuss'.

Some appeared to have come to terms with their fears, as reflected in the following comments:

> *A lot of my friends say, 'how can you do that job, are you not scared about doing that job...?' It's quite a valid point, but because we are used to it, we've become immune to it. Someone's got to do it.*

The midwives from outside London expressed less fear of infection:

> *I'd be a bit upset... but there's nothing you can do until you've actually got your results.*

Some midwives acknowledged having had blood splashes to their eyes. One inner London midwife felt her risk from this was quite high, stating, 'it's as if you are injecting yourself'.

There was general agreement that they were not at risk of becoming infected from exposure of blood to their intact skin. There was also an acknowledgement of the risk of infection when a small cut or break in skin was not covered with a plaster.

Evidence of discriminatory practice

This study confirms the findings of previous studies which identified that some healthcare workers, particularly those working in a low HIV prevalence area, attempt to determine whether or not the patient is in a 'high risk' category and adopt infection control measures accordingly (Bauer and Kenney, 1993; Henry *et al*, 1992). Henry *et al* (1992), who conducted their research in a low HIV prevalence area, reported that healthcare workers attempt to determine which patients are likely to be infected and exercise discriminate caution in their use of barrier protection, for example. This study confirms that the midwives who were practising in a low HIV prevalence area (outside London) were less likely to wear gloves when taking blood from women or when obtaining blood for newborn blood spot screening. Also, they were less likely to wear gowns, and none wore eye protection or protective footwear when assisting a woman who was giving birth. They did, however, advocate the use of barrier protection when taking blood from a woman who was considered to be 'high risk', and they appeared to exercise discriminatory practice when assisting women who were giving birth, as reflected in the following statement:

> *If I was delivering somebody who was HIV or hepatitis B positive, I think, just naturally, you would take greater precautions. I might even put a gown on for instance.*

In contrast, the midwives in inner London treated all women the same, as reflected by the following comments:

> *Because you never know, we can't make assumptions.*
> *We cannot differentiate between someone who might look the part.*
> *You shouldn't really judge people just by their appearance.*

One midwife did, however, raise the possibility of wearing a mask if the lady was known to be HIV positive.

Barriers to the adoption of UP

Several factors appeared to act as barriers to the adoption of UP by practising midwives. The following factors identified by the midwives confirm the findings of other studies:

- lack of time when coping with an emergency (Bauer and Kenney, 1993; Schillo and Reischl, 1993)
- poorly fitting gloves and/or gowns (Bauer and Kenney, 1993; Schillo and Reischl, 1993)
- gloves and/or gowns that leak (Bauer and Kenney, 1993)
- gloves that interfered with the healthcare worker's ability to perform procedures (Bauer and Kenney, 1993; Saghafi *et al*, 1992; Gershon *et al*, 1995; Schillo and Reischl, 1993)
- barrier protection that was awkward or poorly constructed (Schillo and Reischl, 1993).

These were all factors that appeared to make staff less likely to adopt UP.

Interference with performing procedures

Barrier protection often fitted poorly, and interfered with the midwives' ability to carry out procedures, such as venepuncture or undertaking a newborn blood spot screening. Problems with wearing gloves were elaborated as follows:

If the gloves don't fit properly, you can't do it. You just have to be careful.

If the gloves are a large size, it's impossible, because you're trying to grab the glove which is hanging off you and do the procedure at the same time.

You can't feel properly through the gloves... you get wrinkles on your fingers and you're meant to be finding a vein.

Difficulties were also experienced when goggles 'steamed up', which could be exacerbated by wearing masks.

Uncomfortable/impractical/inadequate

The midwives said that they became extremely hot wearing gowns, plastic aprons, masks and overshoes. When wearing gauntlets for water births, midwives with small arms found that water seeped down through the top of the gauntlet due to the tops not fitting properly.

Goggles were found to fit poorly and sometimes fell off. They were 'cumbersome', particularly when worn over prescription glasses.

The wearing of overshoes was also seen to be impractical. One midwife asked, 'are you meant to take them off when you leave the delivery suite — if you've got to pop out and get something, and put them on again?' Another midwife said that they split easily.

Some midwives commented that the gowns were not completely waterproof, causing uncertainty about how to protect themselves effectively. One midwife concluded that gauntlets should be worn when rupturing the membranes.

Perception that barrier protection was detrimental to the midwives' safety or unnecessary

The wearing of overshoes had caused midwives to slip. One midwife said, 'I think they'd be a bit dangerous really'. They were seen to be unnecessary by some midwives, as reflected in the following statement: 'what infection would you get through your shoes from the floor?'

Similarly, poorly fitting gloves were seen to be detrimental to midwives' safety, as reflected in the following statements:

You might actually end up doing more injury to yourself with those gloves that are there.

It would be interesting to do a study to see if there are more needlestick injuries when people wear gloves.

Some midwives felt the wearing of gowns was unnecessary. For example, one said she felt adequately protected wearing a plastic apron, which covered her 'from head to toe'. Another felt that the gloves were long enough to protect her arms.

Lack of time

Lack of time sometimes contributed to the problem of adopting UP. Midwives were less likely to protect themselves adequately when coping with emergencies. For example, when managing a postpartum haemorrhage, one midwife admitted exposing herself to 'quite a bit of risk'. In such cases gloves would always be worn, but the midwives would be unlikely wear an apron. One midwife said, 'by the time you've got yourself kitted out in this... the baby's out'.

Workload also affected the amount of time midwives could take to clean blood spillage (using granules) effectively:

> *I'm sorry, but... we are so busy that you don't stand there and think about it. I need the room, so I'm just going to have to clear it up. That's reality. That's a fact. I would love the granules to stay longer, but if there is someone outside waiting for the room, then I have to clear it up as best I can.*

Perception that barrier protection adversely affects women's birth experience

From a managerial perspective, the UP policy was described as being 'user-friendly' by the manager from inner London because it had been introduced 'gently'. This argument was elaborated as follows:

> *Instead of wearing 'big, huge visors', 'nice glasses' are being worn.*

> *I am distancing myself from the women by wearing protective attire, but we are using 'user-friendly specs'.*

She concluded:

> *I think we've got it right, wearing aprons, gowns, specs, gloves, which feels 'normal'.*

However, the midwives from outside London felt the adoption of UP was not in keeping with the concept of normal childbirth. They felt the wearing of gowns and goggles would conflict with the need to create a 'homely environment' and the development of a trusting relationship with the women. The following comments reflect these attitudes:

If you're gowned-up and goggled and what not, you're creating barriers. It's not quite as relaxing and homely. It's not quite 'with women', is it really?'

If somebody insists you wear goggles and gowns it breaks down that relationship that somebody could have built up during a normal event.

I think that's abysmal, unless the lady's got malaria or something. I'd be frightened if someone came into me dressed like that. You'd be thinking, 'what are they going to do to me?'

I think the mother would probably feel that she had got something, when the midwife puts on all this protection.'

The midwives from both inner and outer London seemed unanimous in their response to the photograph of a midwife wearing a plastic visor to protect the eyes and upper part of the face, and a facemask covering the mouth.

It would aggravate me — because you have to give the mother so much verbal support and encouragement — how can you talk through all that — you'd get so hot and bothered.

That's a bit over the top.

This is more or less like you are working in a Foundry.

Midwives' autonomy

The manager from outside London pointed out that midwives are autonomous practitioners who have a right to choose whether or not they adopt UP. Presumably, because they were practising in a part of the country with a low HIV prevalence among pregnant women, the manager felt the midwives adopted the approach 'it doesn't affect us, so why should we worry?'

Factors which motivated midwives to adopt UP

The following factors appeared to have motivated the midwives to adopt UP.

Concern for their family

Some midwives felt that adopting UP indirectly protected their families. For example, one midwife commented that putting herself at risk could affect her future family or anyone else 'down the line from yourself'. Another commented, 'I don't want to take anything home to the family'.

Recognition of women's need for protection

It was felt that a policy of UP was reassuring for women who may be concerned about their own safety and need for protection from infection. One midwife justified the need to adopt UP 'because she doesn't know what I've got'.

Perception of risk

Awareness of the HIV prevalence rate among pregnant women appeared to act as a stimulus for the adoption of UP. This was evident as the inner London manager pointed out the importance of a UP policy, bearing in mind the local prevalence of HIV among pregnant women was 1 in 200.

The midwives' perception of their risk of occupational infection, and their awareness of the need to adopt UP, had developed as a result of attending lectures and study days, the media, and reading. As one midwife from inner London commented, 'you know it's real — everybody knows this is happening'.

Conducive work environment

The following factors contributed to a conducive work environment:

- key hospital personnel were instrumental in developing the midwives' understanding and providing a supportive network for the implementation of UP. These included the HIV counsellor (inner London), members of the infection control team, and the head of bacteriology (outside London)
- equipment availability
- working with colleagues who were already adopting UP
- posters on display in the sluice and by sharps containers. These reinforced health and safety practice issues, eg. avoiding re-sheathing needles, dealing with blood spillages and managing exposure incidents such as eye splash and needlestick injuries
- well-planned and publicised guidelines for UP
- recent implementation of routine HIV screening for pregnant women.

Hospital policy

One factor that appeared to motivate the inner London midwives to adopt UP was associated with what was described as 'defensive practice'. They were discussing whether all midwives, including those who wore prescription glasses should wear goggles. They agreed that they should be worn because of the hospital policy. One midwife argued:

> *If there is an accident, the authority is going to say, 'look, glasses or no glasses, you should have protected yourself'.*

The implication that midwives should wear goggles over prescription glasses did, however, cause some giggling.

Further comments, which reflect the way in which hospital policy motivated midwives to adopt UP include:

> *If you don't wear it, it's provided — so if you don't wear it, it's on your head, isn't it! — so why not?*

> *If you have sustained a needlestick injury or a puncture wound... I don't think you would have any comeback if (a) you were not wearing gloves, or (b) you didn't have any apron on, or didn't adhere to safety practices, ie. not re-sheathing needles.*

The effectiveness and accessibility of the hospital policy appeared to reflect the extent to which UP were adopted. For example, in inner London where UP were more widely adopted, the UP policy was accessible to all midwives, and guidelines were also available. However, outside London, where UP were less frequently adopted, the hospital policy needed reviewing. For example, the wearing of goggles was not specified in the policy, and the manager said that individual midwives were left to make their own decisions in relation to how they adopted UP in practice.

Managerial issues

From a managerial perspective, several factors appeared to facilitate effectively the adoption of UP by the midwives.

Teamworking

The degree to which UP were adopted appeared to correlate with the way in which 'team players' worked together. For example, having identified the need to change the working environment from one which was described as potentially dangerous, to one which was safer, the inner London manager networked with the senior infection control nurse, the HIV counsellor and the theatre manager to change slowly the environment and implement a UP policy. Also, there were plans for the infection control team to audit the working environment to enable the midwifery managers outside London to take appropriate action.

The inner London manager also stressed the importance of team working together with the midwives. For example, the midwives were encouraged to consider the best interests of others by making sure that the sharps containers were never left over-full for the next person to use. This was described as 'caring about each other'.

Provision of protective attire/equipment

Managerial responsibility involved balancing the budgetary allowance with the need to provide the best possible protective attire and equipment. Protective attire included good quality, low allergy 'Biogel' gloves. Although more expensive, they had a low breakage rate, and fitted well, particularly around the wrist. Latex gloves were also provided. These were cheaper and could be used for changing incopads. Waterproof gowns were randomly tested for permeability, and green plastic gowns were provided for wearing underneath waterproof gowns as a 'back-up'. Goggles and overshoes were also provided for staff to wear during procedures involving risk of blood or body fluid exposure.

The provision of equipment included vacutainers and disposable equipment, such as speculums. In addition, the manager from inner London was considering the feasibility of providing 'tyre' disposal drapes, for use during caesarean sections. They would enable blood and amniotic fluid to collect in the 'tyre', as opposed to dripping onto the floor and footwear of the staff working in theatre. Other practices were also being considered, such as using blunt, as opposed to 'taper-cut' needles for suturing.

Monitoring safety standards

Managerial responsibility involved monitoring safety in the workplace. For example, the inner London manager regularly monitored the sharps disposal containers and placenta buckets to ensure that they were not being over-filled. If any such hazards were observed, the midwives concerned were reminded of the importance of individual members of staff taking responsibility to ensure the working environment is a safe place for all members of staff.

Managing exposure incidents

The reporting and management of exposure incidents varied between the two hospitals. The inner London manager took responsibility for ensuring that staff were aware of the importance of reporting all exposure incidents. Midwives were encouraged to reflect on their practice following a needlestick injury or eye splash. This involved examining what had happened, and discussing whether things could have been done differently to prevent further incidents from re-occurring in the future. Details of the incident, for example, why goggles had not been worn, would be noted on the incident form. The midwives appeared to be familiar with reporting the incident to their manager and filling in an incident form.

Following a needlestick injury, the manager and the midwife concerned would discuss the incident with the source patient, and the HIV counsellor would discuss HIV testing. The HIV counsellor would also liaise with the occupational health staff, and the midwife would be offered antiretroviral therapy. Should the source patient refuse HIV testing, the midwife concerned would be advised to have a follow-up blood test for HIV antibodies. If the source patient was found to be HIV positive, she would be informed of the result by the HIV counsellor who would provide post-test counselling.

According to the manager from outside London, some staff failed to report exposure incidents, and the manager commented that it was difficult to make staff comply with reporting procedures. Instead of reporting exposure incidents to their manager, the midwives said they went to casualty where 'various forms would be filled in, and the midwife would have her blood tested'. They also said the midwife would need a further blood test six months later to assess for seroconversion.

Training

Although both of the managers acknowledged the relevance of staff training when implementing UP, there were differences between the two hospitals as to how this was provided. The inner London hospital provided regular training sessions on UP, which were attended by all midwives. The HIV counsellor was responsible for organising the programme, during which the midwives were able to discuss UP in practice and implementation of the policy. The infection control nurse was also involved in implementing the training.

The hospital outside London did not have a specific training programme to support the implementation of UP. However, weekly 'in-service' education sessions were held to keep the midwives updated on a variety of practice issues, which could include 'health and safety issues'. Regular staff appraisals were conducted, and, if awareness in relation to UP was highlighted as being a problem, individual staff development would be planned accordingly. This would involve sending the midwives on an appropriate study day, or directing them to the relevant hospital policies.

Discussion

The finding that midwives do not always adopt UP or dispose of needles safely confirms the findings of the studies referred to earlier in this chapter, which examined healthcare workers' practice in relation to UP (Hersey and Martin, 1994; Bauer and Kenney, 1993; Henry *et al*, 1992). In addition, a further study, known as the 'HIV/AIDS and Midwifery Project', supports my finding that midwives do not always adequately protect themselves (Grellier *et al*, 1996). The researchers used focus group discussions and self-completion questionnaires to gather data from 336 midwifery students, 98 tutors and 51 midwives from all the midwifery colleges within the South Thames region, and one hospital in a higher HIV prevalence area and two hospitals in a lower HIV prevalence area. Over 30% of student midwives and approximately 60% of practising midwives reported having been exposed to blood and body fluids during the course of their practice. The most frequently reported exposures were needlestick injuries and splashes of body fluids to the face, eyes or mouth, often during the birth of a baby.

In my study, the assistant moderator noted that, generally, the midwives from inner London appeared to be very honest about their practice. She did, however, feel that they appeared to be slightly anxious about 'saying the right things'. It was noted that the laughter at certain points sometimes gave this impression. She also noted that there was a tendency for a midwife to look sideways at me, smiling, as if to say, 'I'm saying this because I should be saying it'. This was an interesting observation, which suggests that the midwives from inner London were less compliant in their adoption of UP than the findings convey.

The term 'defensive practice' was used by one midwife to sum up the general feeling that UP should be adopted because 'the authority' says 'you should have protected yourself'. This is a new finding. Although I tried to reduce the possibility of influencing the responses throughout the research process, it is possible that 'going native' caused the midwives to exaggerate their compliance with UP. Aware of the fact that I was a senior lecturer in midwifery, they may have consciously or sub-consciously perceived me as representing an 'authority figure'. Various problems have been associated with 'going native', and Spradley (1979) and Davies (1995) have warned that ethnographers should always consider the effect that they have upon their informants.

At one point, I was asked to clarify the correct procedure for managing needlestick injury. I gave a non-committal response, reiterating that I was interested in hearing their views. Although the midwives were aware of my status, I endeavoured to ensure that I was non-directive when facilitating the discussion. Objectivity was further enhanced, as neither the assistant moderator nor myself had previously worked in the two hospitals, either as midwives or as clinical liaison lecturers.

The assistant moderator noted that some midwives were hearing concepts such as, 'you don't bleed the wound if you've got a needlestick injury' for the first time, and they were asking each other, 'what do we do here?'

Some of the midwives appeared to be uncertain about what was the best practice, for example, when a midwife reported her needlestick injury to the occupational health sister. It is essential that updated guidelines for best practice are communicated to all healthcare professionals. Failure to address such issues contributes to confusion and uncertainty. My findings highlight the importance of teamworking within the hospital, and guidelines that are easily accessible, universally accepted, and based upon the best available evidence at that time.

The finding that midwives, as autonomous practitioners, sometimes question the need to comply fully with the adoption of UP is also new. For example, many midwives questioned the need to wear protective footwear. Some of the midwives, mainly those practising outside London, also questioned the need to wear waterproof gowns when assisting women who were giving birth. Instead, they preferred to wear plastic aprons, arguing that if any blood did come into contact with their bare arms, the skin would act as a barrier to infection. The assistant moderator also questioned the need to wear waterproof gowns. She believed the midwives from inner London lacked understanding of the skin acting as a barrier to HIV infection, and argued that the need to protect the arms from blood or body fluids was unrealistic. She also maintained that the decision to avoid blood exposure to the arms should be a personal decision, made by the individual midwife in relation to her own practice.

This questioning attitude is not surprising, particularly as, according to Gerberding *et al* (1995), no randomised study has ever shown that the adoption of UP by healthcare workers reduces the risk of HIV transmission. The use of UP should, however, be recognised as good practice. Such practice ensures that any small cracks in the skin, which may be barely visible to the naked eye, are prevented from becoming a potential route for occupational transmission of HIV infection.

MCE accounted for 22% of the 1800 occupational exposures to bloodborne viruses in healthcare workers reported to the Health Protection Agency's, Communicable Disease Surveillance Centre Enhanced Surveillance Programme from 1 July 1997 to 30 June 2003. According to the six-year report, entitled *Surveillance of Significant Occupational Exposure to Bloodborne Viruses in Health Care Workers* (in England, Wales and Northern Ireland) (Health Protection Agency, 2004a), percutaneous injury, the majority of which involved a hollowbore needle was the most commonly reported type of exposure [71%] (1282/1800). The report states that a significant number of these exposures were preventable with adherence to UP and safe disposal of clinical waste. Exposure incidents occurred most frequently on the ward (44% of reported incidents). Fifty-eight per cent of all exposures occurred during a procedure, mainly as a result of the patient moving or becoming agitated. However, some exposure incidents were due to re-sheathing needles, the sharp item being left on the bed or floor, the use of inappropriate waste containers, and items protruding from, or piercing disposal containers. The report states that these occurrences may be minimised by adopting a safer working environment, and highlights the importance of training for healthcare workers to enable them to adopt 'good practice'.

My research findings demonstrate that a conducive work environment appears to motivate midwives to adopt 'good practice'. In particular, posters on display in the clinical areas reminded the midwives of good practice. The Health Protection Agency has produced a poster, *First Aid for Health Care Workers* (Health Protection Agency (2004b) (*Figure 5.1*) which is available online. The poster is a useful reminder to staff of action to be taken following exposure incidents, and it also provides contact details for further information.

In addition, midwives who were already adopting UP in practice contributed to the creation and maintenance of a conducive work environment. Social learning theorists have developed a body of knowledge which supports the concept of learning through observation, or watching the behaviour of others (Gross, 1990). People learn through observing other role models in a particular setting. Initially, UP was a new concept in midwifery practice, but gradually the midwives from inner London became more accustomed to using UP through observing others wearing the protective attire, and interacting with the work environment.

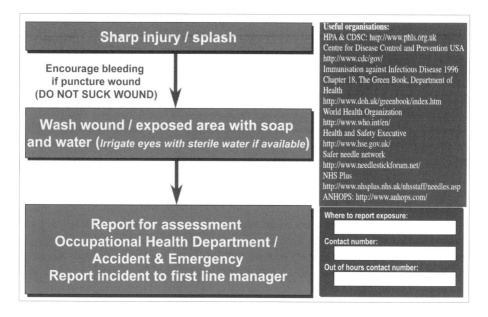

Figure 5.1: First aid for healthcare workers

My recommendations for introducing effective change into the working environment would include using role models. This could operate at two levels. From a managerial level, a manager wishing to facilitate effective implementation of UP could visit another hospital, for example, in inner London, where the policy is being more actively implemented, as demonstrated by my findings, and 'shadow' one of the managers to learn, through observation, aspects of managerial effectiveness in relation to UP. Secondly, key midwives could be identified within the practice areas who could function as role models to other midwives within the area. These midwives would have undertaken initial and ongoing training, and would be committed to seeing UP effectively implemented within the clinical setting. As such, they would be recognising the need to show a duty of care and responsibility towards other midwives, in terms of helping to make the clinical setting a safer environment within which midwives can work.

Gerberding *et al* (1995) feel that one of the main problems in relation to UP, is the fact that a great deal of effort and expense is being focused on an area that does not account for the majority of HIV transmission. They argue that as 85% of the transmission of HIV to healthcare workers is through needlestick injury, more attention should be directed to developing devices, such as self-capping needles, and devices that allow one-handed re-capping of needles, to prevent the possibility of needlestick injury. My research has shown that managerial commitment to introducing safer devices and equipment is beneficial for improving the safety of the work environment. For example, the interest in introducing 'tyre drapes' and blunt needles.

According to my findings, several factors acted as barriers to the adoption of UP by midwives, and other studies have reported similar findings. For example, Grellier *et al* (1996) reported that midwives often regard UP as impractical, obstructive or pointless. In common with the midwives in my study, the midwives in their study were concerned about the risk of occupational infection, and there was a pervasive belief that precautions should be taken. However, the findings of my study identify alternative ways in which midwives have adapted their practice to reduce their risk of occupational infection when the recommended precautions were found to be impractical. For example, one midwife talked about milking the cord before cutting it.

The midwives in my study also referred to leaving perineal tears to heal spontaneously, thereby avoiding suturing. Research findings support this practice as being beneficial to women. Researchers in Sweden compared eighty term pregnant primiparas with minor perineal lacerations of grades I–II who were randomised after childbirth (Lundquist *et al*, 2000). The experimental group (n=40) was non-sutured and the control group (n=40) was sutured. Women were entered into the trial if they met the conditions displayed in *Table 5.1*:

The study failed to demonstrate any significant differences in the healing process, although the sutured group visited the midwife more often because of discomfort from the stitches. Sixteen per cent of the women in the sutured group, but none in the non-sutured group considered that the laceration had had a negative influence on breast-feeding. The researchers concluded that minor perineal lacerations can be left to heal spontaneously. Benefits for the woman include avoiding the discomfort of anaesthesia and suturing, and providing a positive affect on breast-feeding. Benefits for the midwife include more time to focus on supporting breast-feeding, and reduced risk of PCE.

Table 5.1: Inclusion criteria for minor lacerations (Lundquist *et al*, 2000)	
Labia minora	Laceration should not bleed; labia not to be ripped apart
Vagina	Laceration should not bleed and the edges should fall well together; the mucus should not be completely separated from the bottom of the vagina
Perineum	Laceration should not bleed; laceration edges should fall well together when the woman puts her legs together; the depth and length of the laceration should not exceed 2cmx2cm

The midwives in my study who worked in an area of low HIV prevalence (outside London) were concerned that the adoption of UP would conflict with the need to create a 'homely environment' and with the development of a trusting relationship with a woman during labour. Grellier *et al* (1996), also discovered that midwives were concerned about wearing barrier precautions, particularly eye protection, which they believed adversely affected their relationship with the women. They reported:

> *Midwives frequently described their relationship with clients as 'intimate' and believed that eye protection created a barrier which would destroy this intimacy.*

Further research would help to confirm whether this is a correct assumption. As one of the midwives in my study from inner London commented, 'when a woman is pushing, she probably wouldn't be bothered what the midwife was wearing'. Furthermore, one of the midwives pointed out that many women feel reassured to see midwives wearing protective attire, which is seen as 'good practice'.

Failure to implement effectively the adoption of UP by midwives may lead to midwives stereotyping certain women, resulting in discriminatory practice. My findings support this notion. For example, the midwives outside London were unlikely to wear gloves when taking blood from a woman, although they agreed that they would wear gloves if the woman was in a 'high risk' category for HIV infection. One of the midwives said:

> *If I was delivering somebody who was HIV... I think... you would take greater precautions. I might even put a gown on for instance.*

Grellier *et al* (1996) found that although midwives acknowledged the need to wear glasses and gowns for deliveries, they often categorised clients according to their appearance or according to whether they were African. This would affect whether or not they wore the full protective barriers. Such discriminatory practice may be upsetting for the women concerned.

According to my findings, various factors appeared to motivate midwives to adopt UP. An awareness of these factors may assist managers and educators to enable midwives to adopt good practice. One factor that appeared to motivate the midwives was their perception of risk. My findings suggest that information on the local HIV prevalence among pregnant women should be included in educational programmes, as this is beneficial in developing midwives' understanding of their perception of risk.

Effective educational programmes should enable midwives to reflect upon and evaluate their practice to develop good practice. My findings indicate that some midwives, particularly those working in high HIV prevalence areas, were frightened of becoming infected with HIV. This finding has been confirmed by Grellier *et al* (1996), who found that of the ninety-nine midwives who completed their questionnaires, 16% were very worried about the possibility of occupational transmission of HIV, 78% were slightly worried, and 24% were not worried. Midwives would therefore benefit from educational programmes that provide opportunity for fears to be expressed and addressed.

The process of analysing the research data involves demonstrating links to enhance critical understanding of the research problem through the use of visual symbolic representations. A diagrammatic representation has been designed with this in mind. *Figure 5.2* contains an inner circle which represents the practising midwife's adoption of UP. This can be compared to the sun which is part of a complex solar system. A hoop, representing the factors that motivate the midwife to adopt UP is suspended around this inner circle. This may be compared to different planets orbiting the sun. The arrows, radiating from the planets and pointing towards the sun, represent the various forces or motivating factors which are identified as 'straplines'. Another wider hoop containing other planets is suspended further away from the sun. The arrows linking the midwife and this hoop are pointing away from the midwife, in the opposite direction, to represent opposing forces or barriers to the adoption of UP, which are identified in the 'straplines' adjacent to the arrows.

Williams *et al* (1994) suggest that healthcare workers weigh up the obstacles to compliance with UP against the possible benefits. If midwives perceive the benefits of adopting UP as outweighing the barriers, they are more likely to be compliant in their adoption of UP. My research has shown that the midwives who worked in a low HIV prevalence area perceived that the obstacles outweighed the perceived benefits, and this was reflected in their lack of compliance in adopting UP.

By applying the 'Health Belief Model', first described in 1974 by Rosenstock, Williams *et al* (1994) explain how individual healthcare workers have beliefs or fears that they are personally vulnerable to disease. This has been termed 'perceived susceptibility', or the perceived likelihood of acquiring the disease. In addition, the 'perceived seriousness' of the situation is considered, as the healthcare worker assesses the possibility of illness and death, and the perceived impact of the disease on their job, their health and their relationships. Since the introduction of post-exposure prophylaxis for healthcare workers following significant exposure to HIV-infected blood or body fluids, midwives may feel less vulnerable to the possibility of occupational infection.

The hoops which represent the two opposing forces in *Figure 5.2* may be different for different groups of midwives. For example, for a midwife practising outside London, the inner hoop would represent factors that act as barriers to the midwife's adoption of UP (*Figure 5.3*). This hoop is closer to the centre to signify that the force of the barriers to the adoption of UP is likely to be stronger than the force of the motivating factors, which are represented in the outer hoop. This midwife would be less likely to adopt UP in practice. Conversely, *Figure 5.1* may be more representative of a midwife practising in inner London, where the motivating factors could outweigh the barriers to the adoption of UP.

To complete the picture, a rocket has been assigned to reach the sun. This represents managerial support to encourage the adoption of 'good practice' by midwives. Aspects of effective support include provision of training , fostering team working, provision of protective attire and equipment, monitoring safety standards and managing exposure incidents.

Conclusions

Qualitative research was undertaken to assess and develop the adoption of UP in midwifery practice. My findings suggest that although midwives generally recognise the need to adopt UP, this belief is not always translated into practice. The midwives working in inner London were more likely to express fear of infection, and were more likely to adopt UP. There was some evidence of discriminatory practice, particularly among those midwives working outside London.

During the focus group discussions, various areas of ambiguity and confusion were identified in relation to the practice of UP. Failure to adopt UP may result in significant occupational exposure to bloodborne viruses. Various strategies for reducing their risk of exposure were identified by the midwives, sometimes as an alternative to adopting the recommended UP.

Various barriers were identified, that interfered with the adoption of UP in practice. In addition, factors that motivated the midwives to adopt UP were apparent, and managerial support appeared to have a positive affect on the extent to which the midwives adopted 'safe practice' (see *Figures 5.1* and *5.2*).

The following recommendations highlight some key points.

Recommendations

- ⌘ Effective education should be provided to support the adoption of UP by midwives. Educational provision should include training to ensure all midwives know how to use vacutainers, information regarding HIV prevalence among pregnant women, discussion of 'safe practice' and post-exposure prophylaxis, and opportunities for midwives to reflect on practice.
- ⌘ Evidence-based guidelines which reflect current DoH recommendations should be available to reduce the possibility of confusion and ambiguity regarding best practice.
- ⌘ Implementation of updated guidelines should be included in training programmes for midwives.
- ⌘ Managers should monitor the effectiveness of barrier protection, for example, ensuring that gowns are waterproof.
- ⌘ Managers should introduce newly-engineered devices as they become available.
- ⌘ Managers should network with other personnel, for example, the HIV counsellor and the infection control team.
- ⌘ Teamworking should be encouraged, for example, every midwife should take responsibility for changing the sharps containers when necessary.
- ⌘ Managers should seek to encourage a conducive work environment that supports the adoption of UP by midwives. This may be achieved through displaying posters in key places and providing good quality barrier protection in a variety of sizes, as appropriate, to ensure the best possible fit. Protective attire, equipment, sharps disposal containers and guidelines should be easily accessible in the work place.
- ⌘ Key midwives should be identified to act as role models, and to encourage the promotion of safe practice.
- ⌘ Clear guidance should be made available to ensure appropriate management of exposure incidents. Managers should encourage reflection on practice to consider how such occurrences might be prevented in future practice.

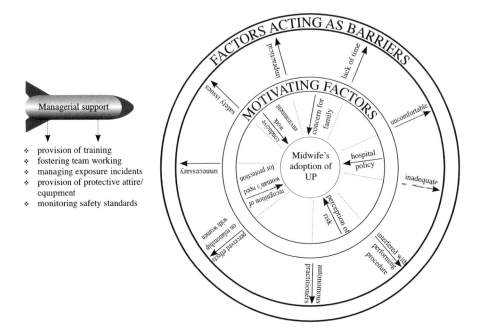

Figure 5.2: A diagrammatic representation of the midwife's adoption of UP (practising inside London)

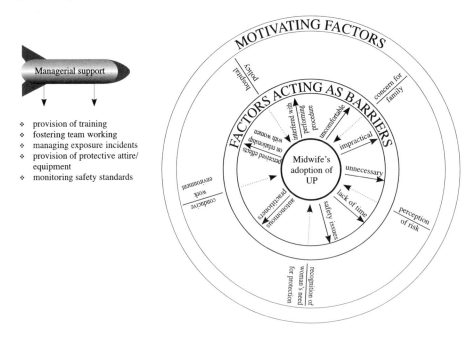

Figure 5.4: A diagrammatic representation of the midwife's adoption of UP (practising outside London)

References

Atkinson P (1979) Research design in ethnography. Block 3. In: Evans J, Sapsfored RJ, eds. *Research Design*. Open University Press, Milton Keynes

Bauer BJ, Kenney JW (1993) Adverse exposures and use of universal precautions among perinatal nurses. *J Obstet Gynaecol Neonat Nurs* **22**(5): 429–35

Centers for Disease Control and Prevention (1985) Transmission of infection with human T-lymphadenopathy-associated virus in the workplace. *Morb Mortal Wkly Rep* **34**: 681–6, 691–5

Centers for Disease Control and Prevention (1987) Recommendations for prevention of HIV transmission of human immunodeficiency virus in health care settings. *Morb Mortal Wkly Rep* **36**(s2):1–37

Centers for Disease Control and Prevention (1988) Update: universal precautions for prevention of transmission of human immunodeficiency virus, hepatitis B and other bloodborne pathogens in health care settings. *Morb Mortal Wkly Rep* **37**: 377–88

Centers for Disease Control and Prevention (1989) Guidelines for the prevention of transmission of human immunodeficiency virus and hepatitis B to health care and public safety workers. *Morb Mortal Wkly Rep* **38**(s6):3-37

Davies R (1995) Introduction to Ethnographic Research in Midwifery. *Br J Midwif* **5**(4): 223–7

Department of Health (1998) *Guidance for Clinical Healthcare Workers: Protection Against Infection with Blood-borne Viruses*. Recommendations of the Expert Advisory Group on AIDS and the Advisory Group on Hepatitis. DoH, London

Gerberding JL, Lewis FR, Schecter WP (1995) Are universal precautions realistic? *Surg Clin North Am* **75**(6): 1091–103

Gershon RM, Karkashian C, Felknor S (1994) Universal precautions: an update. *Heart Lung* **23**(4): 352–8

Gershon RM, Vlahov D, Felknor SA, Vesley D, Johnson PC, Delclos GL *et al* (1995) Compliance with universal precautions among health care workers at three regional hospitals. *Am J Infection Control* **23**(4): 225–36

Grellier R, Stears D, Clift S, Clift S, Forrest S (1996) *HIV/AIDS and Midwifery: A study of knowledge, attitudes and practice among midwifery tutors, students and qualified midwives*. Centre for Health Education and Research, Christchurch College, Canterbury. Supported by South Thames Regional Health Authority

Gross RD (1990) *Psychology: The Science of Mind and Behaviour*. Hodder and Stoughton, London

Health Protection Agency (2004a) Surveillance of Significant Occupational Exposure to Bloodborne Viruses in Health Care Workers in England, Wales and Northern Ireland. Six-year Report: March 2004. Available online: http://www.hpa.org.uk/infections/topics_az/bbv/s_report.htm (accessed 17 May, 2004)

Health Protection Agency (2004b) First Aid for Health Care Workers. Available online: http://www.hpa.org.uk/infections/topics_az/bbv/pdf/poster.pdf (accessed 17 May, 2004)

Henry K, Campbell S, Maki M (1992) A comparison of observed and self-reported compliance with universal precautions among emergency department personnel at a Minnesota public teaching hospital: implications for assessing infection control programs. *Ann Emergency Med* **21**(8): 940–6

Hersey JC, Martin LS (1994) Use of infection control guidelines by workers in healthcare facilities to prevent occupational transmission of HBV and HIV: results from a national survey. *Infect Control Hosp Epidemiol* **15**(4): 243–52

Hisrich R, Peters M (1982) Focus groups: an innovative marketing research technique. *Hosp Health Services Administration* **5**: 8–21

Holloway I, Wheeler S (1996) *Qualitative Research for Nurses*. Blackwell Science, Oxford

Hughes D, Dumont K (1993) Using focus groups to facilitate culturally anchored research. *Am J Community Psychol* **21**: 775–806

Kitzinger J (1994) The methodology of focus groups: the importance of interaction between research participants. *Sociol Health and Illness* **16**(1): 103–21

Kitzinger J (1995) Introducing focus groups. *Br Med J* **311**: 299–302

Knafl K, Howard M (1984) Interpreting and reporting qualitative research. *Research Nurs Health* **7**: 17–24

Kreuger A (1994) *Focus Groups. A Practical Guide for Applied Research.* 2nd edn. Sage Publications, London

Kouri DL, Ernest JM (1993) Incidence of perceived and actual face shield contamination during vaginal and caesarean delivery. *Am J Obstet Gynecol* **169**(2): 312–6

Lundquist M, Olsson A, Nissen E, Norman M (2000) Is it necessary to suture all lacerations after a vaginal delivery? *Birth* **27**(2): 79–85

Mariampolski H (1984) The resurgence of qualitative research. *Public Relations J* **40**(7): 21–3

May KA (1991) Interview techniques in Qualitative Research: Concerns and challenges. In: Morse JM, ed. *Qualitative Nursing Research: A contemporary dialogue*. Sage Publications, London

McQuarrie E, McIntyre (1987) What focus groups can and cannot do: a reply to Seymour. *J Product Innovation and Management* **4**: 55–60

Nelsing S, Nielson TL, Neilson JO (1993) Occupational blood exposure among health care workers: II exposure mechanisms and universal precautions: *Scand J Infect Dis* **25**(2): 199–205

Nyamathi A, Shuler (1990) Focus group interviews: a research technique for informed nursing practice. *J Adv Nurs* **15**: 1281–8

Panlilio AL, Welch BA, Bell DM (1992) Blood and amniotic fluid contact sustained by obstetric personnel during deliveries. *Am J Obstet Gynecol* **167**(3): 703–8

PHLS (Public Health Laboratory Service) AIDS, STD Centre at the Communicable Disease Surveillance Centre and Collaborators (1999) Occupational Transmission of HIV. Summary of published data to June 1999. Available online: http:/www.phls.co.uk (accessed 16 August, 2003)

Polit D, Hungler B (1998) *Nursing Research: Principles and methods.* JB Lippincott, Philadelphia

Roane CM (1993) Registered nurses' use of universal barrier precautions in the paediatric emergency room. *Paediatr Nurs* **19**(5): 453–5

Saghafi L, Raselli P, Francillon MD, Francioli P (1992) Exposure to blood during various procedures: results of two surveys before and after the implementation of universal precautions. *Am J Infect Contr* **20**(2): 53–7

Schillo BA, Reischl TM (1993) HIV-related knowledge and precautions among Michigan nurses. *Am J Public Health* **83**(10): 1438–42

Spradley J (1979) *The Ethnographic Interview.* Holt, Rhinehart and Winston, New York

Watts M, Ebbutt (1987) More than the sum of the parts: research methods in group interviewing. *Br Educational Res J* **13**: 25–34

Webb C (1992) The use of the first person in academic writing: objectivity, language and gatekeeping. *J Adv Nurs* **17**: 747–52

Williams CO, Campbell S, Henry K, Collier P (1994) Variables influencing worker compliance with universal precautions in the emergency department. *Am J Infect Control* **22**(3): 138–48

Wilson J, Breedon P (1990) Universal precautions. *J Infect Control Nurs* **86**(37): 67–70

Chapter 6

Health and safety issues

This chapter discusses further health and safety issues for midwives, with reference to relevant Department of Health (DoH) guidelines. Awareness and reflection on practice issues will enable practitioners to reduce their risk of occupational infection to a minimum through the use of risk reduction strategies and post-exposure prophylaxis (PEP). Protection of clients from HIV-infected healthcare workers will also be considered.

Risk reduction strategies

DoH guidelines contain useful information to help healthcare workers protect themselves from occupational infection with blood-borne viruses (DoH, 1998; DoH, 2000). They include risk reduction strategies, which will be discussed in relation to midwifery practice. Risk reduction strategies are of particular relevance in obstetrics where the highest rates of occupational exposure to patients' blood have been recorded (DoH, 1998).

Recommendations include guidelines for staff working in theatre. During caesarean section, special surgical drapes are recommended which act as 'catch basins', preventing blood and amniotic fluid spillage. The use of surgical clips to secure the drapes used in theatre should be avoided. Instead, blunt clips or disposable drapes incorporating self-adhesive film should be used.

Midwives should also take care when suturing perineums to reduce their risk of percutaneous exposure to HIV-infected blood. For example, midwives should tie the suture material using instruments rather than using their fingers. It is also recommended that tissue forceps are used, rather than fingers, for holding tissue while suturing. Student midwives should be taught accordingly.

Despite taking precautions, midwives may inadvertently sustain a needlestick injury. Some midwives may consider wearing double gloves to provide further protection if they are particularly concerned. Double gloves do not prevent sharps injury although wearing double gloves does make the likelihood of inner glove puncture almost six times less likely. In addition, if PCE does occur, it is possible that a reduced volume of blood would be transmitted due to the enhanced wiping effect of the two layers of glove (DoH, 1998). The use of blunt-tipped needles for suturing, where feasible, may reduce the risk of PCE still further (DoH, 1998).

Differences in practice have been found with regard to washing instruments. Some midwives wash the instruments after use, whereas others leave them unwashed (*Chapter 5*). The DoH guidelines (DoH, 1998) recommend that instruments should be washed thoroughly in warm water with detergent, using gloves and protective clothing, before sterilising. The instruments should be washed in warm water because hot water has been found to harden fats, and cold water may cause proteinaceous material to adhere to the instruments.

Most cases of occupationally-acquired HIV have occurred as a result of procedures where a needle or cannula has been inserted into an artery or vein (DoH, 1998). Midwife managers should consider introducing 'safer needle devices' into the practice areas for staff to use, if they are not already being used. Examples of such devices include needles that retract into the syringe after use, those that have a protective shield over the needle, and needleless intravenous systems. There is growing support for tougher action in the UK, as some NHS trusts use a limited number of these new devices that are in everyday use in the USA. Banning the use of traditional needles through legislation could bring a dramatic fall in the number of needlestick injuries, as it has done in America where legislation has been introduced to make 'needle protection' technologies, reporting of needlestick injuries and training for healthcare professionals in sharps' use compulsory (Duffin, 2003).

Some midwives prefer not to wear gloves for venepuncture or when obtaining blood from a baby's heel (see *Chapter 5*). While gloves cannot prevent PCE, they do offer some protection by way of reducing the volume of blood to which the hand is exposed, known as the 'wiping effect' (DoH, 1998). However, the DoH guidelines (DoH, 1998) recognise that midwives who are experienced at performing venepuncture without gloves may prefer not to wear them because of a perceived reduction of manual dexterity and possible consequent increased risk of PCE. While some midwives may choose not to wear gloves for venepuncture, the DoH (1998) advises that gloves should be available to all midwives who wish to wear them. These should be available in a variety of sizes, as poorly fitting gloves may interfere with a midwife's ability to perform procedures (see *Chapter 5*). Studies have shown that if gloves are not the right size, this can act as a barrier for practitioners wearing gloves to protect themselves (Bauer and Kenney, 1993; Schillo and Reischl, 1993). Gloves should conform to the requirements of European Standard 455 (DoH, 1998). Student midwives should be taught to wear gloves for venepuncture while gaining experience. In addition, they should avoid taking blood from women known to be infected with HIV (DoH, 1998).

Risk of transmission

The following factors are associated with an increased risk of occupationally-acquired HIV infection:

- deep injury
- visible blood on the device which caused the injury
- injury with a needle which had been placed in a source patient's artery or vein
- if the source patient has a high viral load, for example, at the time of seroconversion or in the later stages of HIV disease and terminal HIV-related illness (Cardo *et al*, 997; DoH, 2000).

In addition to blood, the following body fluids may pose a risk of HIV transmission if significant occupational exposure occurs (DoH, 2000):

- amniotic fluid
- cerebrospinal fluid
- human breast milk
- pericardial fluid
- peritoneal fluid
- pleural fluid
- saliva in association with dentistry (likely to be contaminated with blood, even when not obviously so)
- synovial fluid
- unfixed human tissues and organs
- any other body fluid if visibly bloodstained
- exudative or other tissue fluid from burns or skin lesions
- semen
- vaginal secretions.

Reporting exposure incidents

Every NHS trust should have developed policies and protocols for reporting and managing exposure incidents (DoH, 1998; DoH, 2000). Surveillance of healthcare workers was initiated in 1984, following the first documented HIV seroconversion from an occupational exposure, which occurred in the UK. Any healthcare worker who has sustained a PCE or a mucotaneous exposure during the course of their work is obliged to report promptly the incident in accordance with the local trust policy. Occupational health departments and genito-urinary medicine (GUM) clinics are encouraged to voluntarily report exposure incidents to the public health laboratory service (PHLS) Communicable Disease Surveillance Centre (CDSC) in England and Wales, or to the Scottish Centre for Infection and Environmental Health (SCIEH) in Scotland (CDSC, 2003). This enhanced confidential surveillance system, launched in July 1997, monitors occupational risk, and the side-effects and benefits of post-exposure prophylaxis. Criteria for inclusion are exposures to HIV, hepatitis C (HCV), hepatitis B (HBV) and where the source status is unknown and the healthcare worker is on PEP. Employers may also be required to report occupational exposure to HIV to the Health and Safety Executive under the Reporting of Injuries, Diseases and Dangerous Occurrences (RIDDOR) Regulations 1995. The reporting of occupational exposure to HIV is normally done when HIV infection, resulting from exposure in the healthcare setting, has occurred (DoH, 2000).

Training

Managers have a statutory duty to provide training in infection control procedures. Such training should ensure that all staff know how to report exposure incidents, and to whom, and that confidentiality would be guaranteed (DoH, 1998). During the training, opportunities should be provided for staff to consider in advance whether, in the event of exposure to HIV, they would wish to take prophylaxis. Examples of scenarios, which provide a useful trigger for discussion are shown in *Box 6.1*.

Management of exposure

Midwives should be aware of the initial action to be taken in the event of a MCE or PCE . All exposure incidents should be reviewed to consider how recurrence might be prevented (DoH, 2000). In the event of a MCE, including an eye splash, which may occur if protective glasses have not been used appropriately, the eye should be irrigated copiously with water, before and after removing any contact lenses. Following a PCE, the site should be washed liberally with soap and water without scrubbing. Antiseptics and skin washes are not recommended as their clinical efficacy has not been demonstrated, and their effect on local defences is unknown (DoH, 2000). Free bleeding of the puncture site should be gently encouraged, avoiding sucking.

PEP is recommended if significant exposure to high risk body fluids known to be or strongly suspected to be infected with HIV has occurred either through:

- needlestick or instrument injury (PCE)
- exposure of broken skin, for example, abrasions, cuts, eczema
- mucous membrane exposure, including eyes (MCE).

Since the introduction of routine screening for HIV during pregnancy, it may be possible to ascertain the HIV status of a woman in the majority of cases. However, if the HIV test result was negative, it may be worth undertaking a 'risk assessment' with the woman in question, as she may have exposed herself to the risk of infection, for example, through unprotected sex with an infected partner since initial testing. The test may need repeating to allow for possible seroconversion which usually takes three months, or sometimes longer. Alternatively, it may be beneficial to consider 'routine' repeat testing, as research suggests that the use of 'risk assessment' is unhelpful. Two studies have shown that when selective screening for HIV was carried out, only 58% (Landesman *et al*, 1987) and 45% (Wemstrom and Zuidema, 1989) of patients identified as being HIV-seropositive had self-identified risk factors. Another large study, which was carried out in an inner-city area of Baltimore in the USA, showed that selective screening of women with identified 'risk factors' would only have detected 57% of HIV-seropositive women.

Box 6.1: HIV — reducing occupational risk scenarios

Scenario 1

While taking blood from a lady at her thirty-four week A/N assessment, you accidentally sustain a needlestick injury. HIV screening at booking had shown no evidence of infection. Discuss the issues raised by this scenario.

Scenario 2

You are providing care to a woman who is progressing well in labour and goes on to have a normal delivery. A student midwife had been allocated to work with you. She is keen to do this delivery, having completed five witness deliveries. Discuss your role in ensuring health and safety in practice during delivery, including immediate care of new-born and placenta-related aspects of care. During the delivery the student did not wear eye protection. Some blood splashed into her eye as she cut the umbilical cord. Discuss the issues raised by this scenario, and the action you would take.

Scenario 3

You are providing care during labour for a woman who is infected with HIV. She has a post-partum haemorrhage following the birth of her baby. Discuss the health and safety issues for reducing occupational risk of infection, including disposal of instruments/needles, dealing with blood spillage and disposal of soiled linen/waste.

Scenario 4

Discuss the precautions taken when suturing the perineum. While suturing the perineum of a lady known to be HIV positive, you inadvertently prick yourself with the blood-stained tip of the suture needle. Discuss effective management of this situation.

By offering counselling and HIV testing to all pregnant women, the detection rate was raised to 87% (Barbacci *et al*, 1991). This may be because women are either unaware of their risk, or they may be unwilling to disclose possible risk factors. Although it is worth considering these issues, the DoH does in fact advise that PEP should not be offered if, on testing, the source patient is shown to be HIV negative, or if risk assessment has concluded that HIV infection of the source is highly unlikely (DoH, 1998).

If testing is being considered, the reasons for testing should be discussed with the source patient. If this is done sensitively, consent is rarely withheld (DoH, 2000). Any midwife who takes blood for testing without consent, or who co-operates in obtaining such a specimen, is liable to face a possible charge of criminal damage or alleged misconduct (UKCC, 1994). The DoH guidelines (1998) state that in exceptional circumstances a doctor may decide to balance the interests of the healthcare worker against those of the source patient and test a blood sample previously taken for other tests. If this were the case, the doctor concerned would need to be able to justify such action.

A midwife should be able to report immediately to designated doctors for information, counselling and psychological support following exposure to potentially infected blood. The midwife may be encouraged to provide a baseline sample of blood for storage, and follow-up samples for testing as appropriate. For example, a healthcare worker exposed to a known HIV positive source should have a baseline serum sample taken, and further samples taken for testing at six, twelve and twenty-four weeks following the exposure incident. If a positive result is reported on any of these occasions then the stored baseline serum would be tested (CDSC, 2003).

Post-exposure prophylaxis

Researchers in the USA have reported that when zidovudine prophylaxis was given to healthcare workers occupationally exposed to HIV, an associated 80% reduction in the risk for occupationally-acquired HIV infection was found (Cardo *et al*, 1997). Combination PEP is now recommended because it is more effective in suppressing viral replication when compared to zidovudine alone. In addition, the increased prevalence of zidovudine resistance among HIV-infected people is becoming more common. The success of PEP has been attributed to the fact that systemic viral dissemination does not occur immediately, leaving a window of opportunity, during which post-exposure antiretroviral medication may be beneficial (DoH, 2000).

Ideally, PEP should be commenced within one hour of the exposure incident, or as soon as possible after the incident. The following drug combinations are recommended:

• zidovudine 200mg three times a day or 250mg twice daily plus

- lamivudine 150mg twice daily plus
- indinavir 800mg three times daily or nelfinavir 750mgs tds/1250mg bd (DoH, 2000).

The advantage of nelfinavir is that it only needs to be taken twice a day, and it need not be taken on an empty stomach. However, it can, cause diarrhoea.

Therapy is continued for four weeks, during which time weekly follow-up is advised to monitor any side-effects of treatment. Prophylactic anti-emetics should also be considered, as nausea is a common problem. Anti-motility drugs may be helpful if diarrhoea develops. In addition to common gastrointestinal side-effects such as nausea and vomiting, malaise, fatigue and headaches can also occur. At least six months should elapse after cessation of PEP before a negative antibody test is used to reassure the midwife that she is infection free.

Occupationally-acquired HIV infection

Figure 6.1 gives details of the total number of healthcare workers with documented and reported HIV seroconversions from an occupational exposure in the UK. All of them sustained percutaneous injuries from hollow-bore devices used in an artery or vein, and all the source patients had high viral loads. Two of the five healthcare workers had received PEP. Unfortunately, four of the five have died and the survival of the one remaining is unknown to the surveillance system (Health Protection Agency, 2003).

Figures 6.2 and *6.3* show the total number of possible HIV occupational acquisitions in the UK. These twelve healthcare workers were diagnosed in the UK, but were occupationally exposed abroad to no other risk for HIV apart from occupational exposure. Three of them are known to have died (Health Protection Agency, 2003).

If, during the six-month follow-up period, seroconversion does occur, an infected healthcare worker may be able to claim Industrial Injuries Disablement Benefit (DoH, 2000). In addition, the NHS Injury Benefits Scheme (or HPSS Injury Benefits Scheme in Northern Ireland) provides temporary or permanent benefits for all NHS employees who lose remuneration because of an injury or disease attributable to their NHS employment.

UK HIV Documented / Reported Occupational Seroconversions (UK 1984 – 2002)

Diagnosis	Occupation	PEP	Exposure	Source Status	First positive
1984	Nurse	No	Resheathing needle	AIDS	Day 49 First +ve
1992-3	Nurse	Yes <1hr	IV cannulation	AIDS	Day 56
1992-3	Phlebotomist	No	Venepuncture	HIV +	Day 90
1992-3	HCW	No	Venepuncture	AIDS	Day 81
1999	Nurse	Yes <90min	Venepuncture	AIDS	Day 90

Enhanced Occupational Surveillance of Bloodborne Viruses July 1997 – July 2002, EW&NI

Source: HARS. CDSC

Figure 6.1: Documented and reported HIV seroconversions from an occupational exposure in the UK

Possible HIV Occupational Acquisition (1) (UK 1984 – 2002)

Diagnosed	Survival	Occupational	Details of Exposure	Possible Acquisition
1988	AIDS '88	Surgeon	Surgery	Africa
1988	AIDS'95	Nurse	Nursing, Midwifery	Africa
1989	?	Nurse	Accident and Emergency	Zambia
1989	?	Nurse Midwife	Midwifery Blood transfusion	Zambia
1992	?	HCW	Healthcare in adverse conditions	Africa

Enhanced Occupational Surveillance of Bloodborne Viruses July 1997 – July 2002, EW&NI

Source: HARS. CDSC

Figure 6.2: Occupational acquisitions of HIV in the UK (Health Protection Agency, 2003)

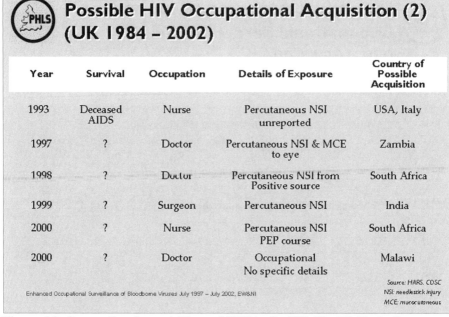

Possible HIV Occupational Acquisition (2) (UK 1984 – 2002)

Year	Survival	Occupation	Details of Exposure	Country of Possible Acquisition
1993	Deceased AIDS	Nurse	Percutaneous NSI unreported	USA, Italy
1997	?	Doctor	Percutaneous NSI & MCE to eye	Zambia
1998	?	Doctor	Percutaneous NSI from Positive source	South Africa
1999	?	Surgeon	Percutaneous NSI	India
2000	?	Nurse	Percutaneous NSI PEP course	South Africa
2000	?	Doctor	Occupational No specific details	Malawi

Enhanced Occupational Surveillance of Bloodborne Viruses July 1997 – July 2002, EW&NI

Source: HARS. CDSC
NSI: needlestick injury
MCE: mucocutaneous

Figure 6.3: Occupational acquisitions of HIV in the UK (Health Protection Agency, 2003)

Protection of the public

The risk of transmission of HIV from a midwife to a patient is far less than the risk of transmission from a patient to a midwife (DoH, 1998). The only two HIV-infected healthcare workers who have been reported as having transmitted HIV infection during exposure-prone procedures were a dentist in Florida, and an orthopaedic surgeon in France (PHLS AIDS and STD Centre at the Communicable Disease Surveillance Centre and Collaborators, 1999). If a midwife suspects that she may have been exposed to HIV infection for any reason, she should seek specialist medical advice and diagnostic testing if applicable (UKCC, 1994). If a midwife is infected with HIV she must take appropriate precautions to prevent transmission of HIV infection to a patient. This would include avoiding exposure-prone procedures where there is a risk that injury to the midwife might result in exposing the patient's open tissue to the midwife's blood, for example, while suturing the perineum. The midwife should be reassigned in such circumstances. An attitude of tolerance towards infected healthcare workers, as opposed to discrimination, is advocated by the Nursing and Midwifery Council (NMC). Hence, midwives should expect a full range of support and strict standards of confidentiality from the Occupational Health Services (UKCC, 1994).

An expert group was set up in 2001 to look at minimising the risks posed to patients from healthcare workers new to the NHS infected with serious communicable diseases, including HIV (DoH, 2003). The final guidance document will be available in due course, as the consultation period has now ended. The proposals are that all new healthcare workers will need to have standard health clearance for serious communicable diseases before appointment or commencement of training. Within the context of reminding new healthcare workers of their professional responsibilities to serious communicable diseases, HIV testing would be offered. During this discussion they should be given a copy of the guidance from the relevant professional regulatory body, for example, from the NMC (DoH, 2003: 29–30) (see *Box 6.2*). Additional health clearance for blood-borne viruses, including HIV, will be needed for new healthcare workers who will perform exposure-prone procedures (DoH, 2003). This would include an 'additional health check' to establish that they are not chronically infected with HIV. Midwifery students would require this additional health clearance as they will be performing perineal suturing during training, as would midwives new to the NHS. Student nurses and nurses new to the NHS would only need standard health clearance. Healthcare workers who apply for a post or training which may involve exposure-prone procedures, and, who decline to be tested for HIV, hepatitis B and hepatitis C should not be cleared to perform exposure-prone procedures.

Conclusion

Midwives can take precautions to protect themselves against occupational transmission of HIV. This involves the use of risk reduction strategies in practice, and being aware of local trust policies for management of exposure incidents. Implementation of such policies should include staff training and reporting procedures in the event of an exposure incident. Training should include opportunities for healthcare workers to consider in advance whether they would wish to take PEP following exposure to blood or body fluids that are infected, or strongly suspected to be infected, with HIV. Midwives also have a duty to protect their patients and should ensure that they adhere to the NMC guidelines for good practice to prevent the transmission of HIV to any patient in their care. Further measures are to be introduced, following the final publication *Health clearance for serious communicable diseases: new healthcare workers* (DoH, 2003). Healthcare workers new to the NHS will have to undergo health clearance for serious communicable diseases. Additional health checks for new healthcare workers who will perform exposure-prone procedures will be required to establish that they are not infected with HIV. Student midwives and new midwives come into this category as the role of the midwife includes perineal suturing.

Box 6.2: United Kingdom Central Council for Nursing, Midwifery and Health Visiting (UKCC) — now the Nursing and Midwifery Council (NMC)

Extract from: Registrar's Letter 4/1994 Annex 1 ACQUIRED IMMUNE DEFICIENCY SYNDROME AND HUMAN IMMUNO DEFICIENCY VIRUS INFECTION (AIDS AND HIV INFECTION) The Council's Position Statement

The Council's *Code of Professional Conduct*

The 'Code of Professional Conduct for the Nurse, Midwife and Health Visitor' is a statement to the profession of the primacy of the interests of patients and clients. Its introductory paragraph states the requirement that each registered nurse, midwife and health visitor safeguard the interest of individual patients and clients. It goes on to indicate to all persons on the register maintained by the Council that, in the exercise of their personal professional accountability, they must 'act always in such a manner as to promote and safeguard the interests and well-being of patients and clients'.

The responsibility of individual practitioners with HIV infection

Although the risk of transmission of HIV infection from a practitioner to a patient is remote, and, on the available evidence much less than the risk of patient to practitioner transmission, the risk must be taken seriously. The Department of Health in England has commissioned a study to evaluate this risk. It is incumbent on the person who is HIV positive to ensure that she or he is assessed regularly by her or his medical advisers and complies with the advice received.

Similarly, a nurse, midwife or health visitor who believes that she or he may have been exposed to infection with HIV, in whatever circumstances, should seek specialist medical advice and diagnostic testing, if applicable. She or he must then adhere to the specialist medical advice received. Each practitioner must consider very carefully their personal accountability as defined in the *Code of Professional Conduct* and remember that she or he has an overriding ethical duty of care to patients.

References

Barbacci M, Repke J, Chaisson R, (1991) Routine prenatal screening for HIV infection. *Lancet* **337**: 709–11

Bauer BJ, Kenney JW (1993) Adverse exposures and use of universal precautions among perinatal nurses. *J Obstet Gynecol Neonatal Nurs* **22**(5): 429–35

Cardo D, Culver DH, Ciesielski CA *et al* (1997) A case control study of HIV seroconversion in health care workers after percutaneous exposure. *N Engl J Med* **337**: 1485–90

Communicable Disease Surveillance Centre (2003) *Surveillance of Occupational Exposure to Bloodborne viruses in healthcare workers.* Five-year report: 1 July 1997 to 30 June 2002

Department of Health (1998) *Guidance for Clinical Healthcare Workers. Protection Against Infection with Blood-borne Viruses. Recommendations of the Expert Advisory Group on AIDS and the Advisory Group on Hepatitis.* HMSO, London

Department of Health (2000) *HIV Post-Exposure Prophylaxis: Guidance from the UK Chief Medical Officers' Expert Advisory Group on AIDS.* DoH, London

Department of Health (2003) Health clearance for serious communicable diseases: new health care workers. Draft guidance for consultation. Available online at: http://www.doh.gov.uk/healthclear/ (accessed 2 October, 2003)

Duffin C (2003) Should traditional needles be banned from the NHS? Available online: http//www.needlestickforum.net/11news/viewstory. asp?NewsID=56 (accessed 10 September, 2003)

Health Protection Agency (2003) Slides for surveillance of occupational exposure to bloodborne viruses in healthcare workers. Available online at: http://www.hpa.org.uk/infections/topics_az/bbv/slides.htm (accessed 22 September 2003)

PHLS AIDS and STD Centre at the Communicable Disease Surveillance Centre and Collaborators (1999) Occupational Transmission of HIV. Summary of published data to June 1999. Available online: http:/www.phls.co.uk (accessed 16 August, 2003)

Landesman S, Minkoff H, Holman S, McCalla S, Sijin O (1987) Serosurvey of HIV infection in parturients. *JAMA* **258**: 2701–3

Schillo BA, Reischl TM (1993) HIV-related knowledge and precautions among Michigan nurses. *Am J Public Health* **83**(10): 1438–42

United Kingdom Central Council for Nursing, Midwifery and Health Visiting (1994) Registrar's Letter 4/1994 Annex 1. Acquired Immune Deficiency Syndrome and Human Immunodeficiency Virus Infection. The Council's Position Statement. UKCC, London

Wemstrom KD, Zuidema LJ (1989) Determination of positive seroprevalence of HIV infection in gravidas by non-anonymous screening. *Obstet and Gynecol* **74**: 558–61

Index

A

acquired immune deficiency syndrome (AIDS) 1
adolescent girls 64
allergic dermatitis 85
amniocentesis 47
amniotic fluid 78–81, 108, 120
anaemia 55
anal squamous intraepithelial neoplasia 26
antibiotics 55
antibodies 49, 51, 56, 62
  maternal 56
antiretroviral therapy 22, 26–28, 32, 34, 43, 46, 48–50, 63, 108
  side-effects of 53
autonomy 42, 57
  midwives' 105

B

bacterial vaginosis 47, 48
barrier protection 80, 82, 85, 86, 94, 95, 101, 103, 104, 117
birth plan 46
blood-stained linen
  disposal of 98
blood spillages 79, 95–98, 104, 106
blood spot screening 95, 101, 102
blood transfusions 55
booking interview 64
bottle-feeding 28, 29, 45
breast-feeding 28, 40, 45, 51
  avoidance of 55
breast milk 55, 78
  virus load 45

British National Survey of Sexual Attitudes and Lifestyles 67

C

caesarean section 28, 47, 54, 81
  elective 46
  RCOG guidelines for elective 47
care
  continuity of 71
certificate of health effect 51
cervical cytological abnormalities 25
cervical intraepithelial neoplasia 26
Changing Childbirth 37
children
  vulnerable 66, 70–74
children's centres 71
child protection 71
Chlamydia trachomatis 31, 47
chorioamnionitis 43
chorionic villus sampling 47
co-trimoxazole 48, 53
colostrum 45
community midwifery services 71
condoms 66, 67
confidentiality 42, 57, 58
  policy 57
confidential surveillance system 124
consent 127
  informed 56, 68
consultant midwives 71
contraception 67
cultural values 88
culture
  mainstream 88
cytomegalovirus (CMV) 24, 25